An Essential Guide to Developing,
Implementing, and Evaluating
Objective Structured Clinical Examination
(OSCE)

An Essential Guide to Developing,
Implementing, and Evaluating
Objective Structured Clinical Examination
(OSCE)

Hamza M. Abdulghani
King Saud University, Saudi Arabia

Gominda Ponnamperuma
Colombo University, Sri Lanka

Zubair Amin
National University of Singapore, Singapore

World Scientific

NEW JERSEY · LONDON · SINGAPORE · BEIJING · SHANGHAI · HONG KONG · TAIPEI · CHENNAI

Published by

World Scientific Publishing Co. Pte. Ltd.

5 Toh Tuck Link, Singapore 596224

USA office: 27 Warren Street, Suite 401-402, Hackensack, NJ 07601

UK office: 57 Shelton Street, Covent Garden, London WC2H 9HE

Library of Congress Cataloging-in-Publication Data
Abdulghani, Hamza M., author.
    An essential guide to developing, implementing, and evaluating Objective Structured Clinical
Examination (OSCE) / Hamza M. Abdulghani, Gominda Ponnamperuma, Zubair Amin.
    p. ; cm.
    Includes bibliographical references and index.
    ISBN 978-9814623520 (hardcover : alk. paper) -- ISBN 9814623520 (hardcover : alk. paper)
    ISBN 978-9814632522 (paperback : alk. paper) -- ISBN 981463252X (paperback : alk. paper)
    I. Ponnamperuma, Gominda, author. II. Amin, Zubair, author. III. Title.
    [DNLM: 1. Clinical Competence. 2. Clinical Medicine--education. 3. Educational
Measurement--methods. WB 18]
    RC58
    616.0076--dc23

                                                                2014028095

British Library Cataloguing-in-Publication Data
A catalogue record for this book is available from the British Library.

Cover illustration by:
Mr. Virgilio I. Salvado
Medical Illustrator
Department of Medical Photography
College of Medicine, King Saud University
Riyadh, Saudi Arabia

FOREWORD

Since its introduction in the 1970s, the Objective Structured Clinical Examination, or OSCE, has become a mainstay of clinical assessment throughout the world. As with any highly successful development, some confusion about its meaning and optimal use has followed its introduction. In particular, a variety of different assessment formats have been called "OSCEs," even though they are not. More frequently, OSCEs have been assembled and used without paying attention to important issues such as blueprinting, standard setting, quality control, and so on. This book takes on the important roles of clarifying the nature of the OSCE and of recommending best practices in terms of its implementation.

In developing the OSCE, Harden *et al.* (1975) were motivated to overcome some of the difficulties of the traditional clinical examination. The traditional clinical evaluation exercise was typically conducted with one patient who was usually in the hospital. A complete history and physical examination was expected of the student, but unobserved. Afterwards, a single examiner, who was familiar with the patient, questioned the student and graded their performance.

This method of assessment had at least three flaws. First, the student was observed with only one patient and there is a significant body of evidence indicating that physician performance is case specific; performance on one case does not predict performance on another, so good assessment requires broader sampling of patients. Second, examiners do not necessarily agree on the quality of a performance even when they are observing exactly the same thing, so broader sampling of examiners is also required. Finally, the traditional clinical evaluation, based on a complete history and physical examination, is unrealistic; doctors rarely spend so much time with a single patient at one visit and most encounters are return visits.

The OSCE was introduced to overcome these flaws. Students rotate through a series of stations, each of which poses a different challenge. The stations tend to be relatively short (5–20 min) and focused on a single task. At one station, the students might face a standardized patient from whom they are required to take a history. At the next, they might perform a procedure or interpret an electrocardiogram. This ensures that the students' assessment is based on a number of different patients or tasks and each of the tasks is realistic.

Students are observed and scored by an examiner when the station warrants it, and he/she typically has a checklist or rating form to complete; the marking is agreed in advance. This ensures that several examiners are involved in the assessment of each student. Further, since students face exactly the same challenges and are judged against the same marking scheme, their scores are directly comparable.

As Ian Hart has noted, the OSCE is *not* a method of assessment. Instead, it is a format within which several different methods of assessment can be organized. So the stations of an OSCE might be composed of real patients, simulated patients, simulations of various types, or some combination of these. In successive chapters, this book presents guidance on which of these methods can and should be used for which purposes. These also serve to underscore one very important source of confusion regarding the OSCE. It is insufficient to describe an examination as an "OSCE" without further describing the methods that are employed as part of it. An OSCE is a format, not a method.

Of course, decisions about which method(s) to use need to be predicated on the purpose of the test, its blueprint or table of specifications, and the test material that is developed. In fact, the quality of the blueprint and the test material are probably the biggest determinants of the meaning and validity of the scores. To signal their importance and provide practical guidance, this book has devoted considerable attention to these important topics that are often ignored in practice.

One area that has engendered considerable confusion regarding OSCEs, as well as other formats of assessment, is scoring and standard-setting. A score is a number or letter that characterizes the correctness of a response or a set of responses. A standard is the score that separates those who pass from those who fail. Often, these two concepts are conflated and/or the judgments supporting them not explicitly separated. This book takes on these two important topics in separate chapters, highlighting the difference between them. In so doing, it melds the latest research and practice experience in providing guidance on how to proceed.

Although the development and scoring of the OSCE have received the most attention, the creation and implementation of quality assurance procedures is important as well. A variety of strategies, many based on double scoring or the analysis of videotapes, can be used to ensure that standardized patients and examiners are well trained. After the fact, it is also possible to use videotapes or other devices to conduct studies aimed at uncovering potential examiner bias, potential standardized patient bias, and differences in examiner stringency. Likewise, it is possible to study and improve the quality of the patient portrayals and to determine how to control their influence on students' scores. These quality assurance mechanisms are essential to good assessment.

Unfortunately, the production of an OSCE can use significant resources. This might be acceptable when those resources are available, but there are a variety of low-income settings where the use of an OSCE is critical to educational quality. It is heartening to see the current authors take on the challenge of these situations and offer practical advice about how to produce an OSCE, even when significant resources are unavailable.

As the OSCE has developed, much emphasis has been put on the use of standardized patient and other forms of simulation. In high-stakes national or regional settings, this makes sense because of the high test volumes and the need for comparable scores.

However, in local settings and particularly in low-resource contexts, the use of real patients has much to recommend it. They offer greater clinical authenticity and can enhance the validity of scores while increasing errors of measurement by only a small extent. This is an area for further research.

Likewise, research and development concerning the OSCE has appropriately focused predominantly on its use as a summative test. Recently, there has been a growing awareness of the role of formative assessment in guiding and creating learning. OSCEs can make a significant contribution to educational quality in this role. However, research is needed in order to determine the optimal use of OSCEs in formative assessment and to determine how to provide feedback based on student performance that maximizes learning.

Finally, individual students have historically been the object of assessment for the OSCE and most other assessment formats. With the growing importance of collaborative learning and practice, the OSCE represents a potential vehicle for both formative and summative assessment in the future. Considerable work is needed, but the flexibility of the OSCE format makes it ideal for exploration in this domain.

The OSCE has changed the way assessment is done. It has ushered in a period when as much educational effort is put into clinical skills as medical knowledge. This book clarifies the meaning of the OSCE and provides advice aimed at ensuring its quality in practice. It is exactly the right time for this contribution.

References

Harden RM, Stevenson M, Downie WW, Wilson GM. (1975) Assessment of clinical competence using objective structured examination. *Br Med J* 1(5955): 447–451.

John J. Norcini Jr. PhD
President and Chief Executive Officer
Foundation for Advancement of International
Medical Education and Research

ACKNOWLEDGMENTS

We are grateful to our students, fellow colleagues, and medical teachers from various parts of the world for providing us with continuous encouragement, stimulation, and learning. We would like to acknowledge the contribution of our medical illustrator, Virgillo J. Salvador from the Department of Medical Photography, College of Medicine, King Saud University, Riyadh, Saudi Arabia.

Hamza Mohammad Abdulghani
Gominda Ponnamperuma
Zubair Amin

PREFACE

Of all the activities that a medical teacher is entrusted to carry out, assessment is perhaps the most critical of all. A student can overcome inadequate teaching from an individual teacher by undertaking their own efforts, but a poorly conducted assessment has a long-lasting effect on the student's learning and competence. More importantly, poor assessment practice undermines the public trust in the medical profession. Therefore, it is imperative that we conduct assessment with the highest possible professional standard.

After many years of relative quiescence, the medical education community has embarked upon embracing clinical assessment as an integral component of the overall assessment of medical students and trainee doctors. Objective Structured Clinical Examination, or OSCE as it is popularly known, has emerged as a practical tool for assessing clinical competencies across the spectrum of medical training — from student selection in a medical school to remediation of trainee doctors, in addition to its more familiar use as a standardized clinical skills examination.

However, within this welcome change, our collective professional observation also suggests that the OSCE has been misused by many. The reasons for this may be varied, but a lack of knowledge about the basic tenants of the OSCE stands out as one of the most important factors, resulting in inappropriate use and implementation of the OSCE as an effective assessment tool. We believe that there is no alternative to faculty training — a sound understanding by the faculty of the fundamental aspects of assessment in general and the OSCE in particular is vital for developing and implementing a robust OSCE.

This book aims to provide a comprehensive overview of the OSCE, from theoretical aspects to practical applications for its appropriate and effective use by medical teachers, medical educators, OSCE planners, clinicians, nursing colleagues, faculty administrators, and others. We present mixed and balanced medical education research and practical tips to provide readers with an easy-to-digest yet comprehensive guide for the implementation of the OSCE. We have started the book with essential theoretical foundations before progressing to practical implementation steps. We have also presented specific topics, such as the OSCE for the selection of candidates and quality assurance, in the later part of the book. For those who want to have a quick answer to their queries, a compilation of frequently asked questions is presented at the end.

We sincerely hope that this book will help you to conceptualize, plan, develop, and implement a robust OSCE to benefit your students and trainees and to safeguard your patients. This is our moral obligation.

CONTENTS

Foreword	v
Acknowledgments	ix
Preface	xi

Chapter 1   The Birth and Propagation of the OSCE 1
The Birth 2
OSCE as a Global Phenomenon 6
Summary 7
References 8

**Chapter 2   The OSCE in the Context of a Holistic
Assessment** 9
How Does the OSCE Fit into
  Overall Assessment? 10
Basic Configuration of an OSCE 12
Why is an OSCE Preferable Over Traditional
  Clinical Examinations? 15
OSCE, Short Cases, and the Mini-CEX 18
OSCE Pretenders or Imitation OSCEs 19
Summary 21
References 21

Chapter 3   Value of the OSCE as an Assessment Tool   23
Validity   24
Reliability   27
Educational Impact   30
Acceptability   33
Cost   34
Summary   34
References   35

**Chapter 4   Selecting the Skills to be Tested in
                an OSCE through Blueprinting   37**
Basic Concepts of Blueprinting   38
Master Blueprint   40
OSCE Blueprint   44
Further Specifications   51
Summary   54
References   54

**Chapter 5   Utilizing Different Formats of OSCE
                for Greater Efficiency   55**
Formative and Summative OSCEs   55
Active and Static Stations   56
Couplet or Linked Stations   58
Long-Station OSCEs   59
Objective Structured Practical Examination   60
Summary   62
References   63

Chapter 6   Writing OSCE Stations   65
Forming the Team to Write the OSCE Station   65
Developing Instructions to the Candidate   66
Developing Instructions to the Simulated
  and Standardized Patients   68
Developing Instructions to the Examiners   71
Preparing Equipment and Materials   73
Summary   76
References   76

**Chapter 7   Creating a Scoring Template
                for Assigning Marks**   77
    Purpose of a Scoring Template   78
    Different Formats of Itemized Checklists   78
    Qualitative Comments   84
    Generic Marking Template   85
    Global Rating   87
    Summary   90
    References   91

Chapter 8   Preparing Patients for the OSCE   93
    Balance between Standardization and Authenticity   95
    Degree of Realism as Portrayed by the Patients   96
    Nature of Tasks to be Tested   98
    Purpose of the OSCE   99
    Logistics and Practical Considerations   100
    Preparing Real Patients for the OSCE   100
    Recruiting and Training Simulated Patients
        for the OSCE   104
    Summary   106
    References   106

**Chapter 9   Preparing Simulators
                for the OSCE**   109
    Simulators and Simulation in Medical Education   110
    Range of Simulators and Simulation   112
    Skills that can be Tested in the OSCE with Simulators   113
    Summary   118
    References   119

**Chapter 10   Preparing the Groundwork for
                Conducting an OSCE**   121
    Faculty Training   121
    Selecting Examiners for an OSCE   123
    Examiners' Briefing   125
    Students' Briefing   127

Pilot Run   127
Checklist for the Day of the OSCE   129
OSCE Administration   130
Security   130
Summary   131
References   131

**Chapter 11   Determining Passes and Fails
              in an OSCE**   **133**
Basic Concepts and Principles of Standard Setting   133
Classical Borderline Group Method
   of Standard Setting   137
Borderline Regression Method   140
Summary   142
References   142

Chapter 12   Post-Assessment Quality Assurance   **143**
Quantitative Data (Item Analysis)   144
Qualitative Data (Feedback)   154
Utilization of Data   156
Summary   156
References   157

Chapter 13   Feedback, Moderation, and Banking   **159**
Feedback to the Curriculum Committee   159
Feedback to the Candidate   160
Moderation of Marks   161
Banking of OSCE Stations   162
Summary   164
References   164

**Chapter 14   Helping Poorly Performing Students
              in an OSCE**   **165**
Importance of Remediation   165
Reasons for Poor Performance in an OSCE   166
Customization of Remediation Strategies   169

Challenges in Remediation   174
Summary   174
References   175

**Chapter 15   OSCE as a Tool for the Selection
                of Applicants**   177
The Flexibility of the OSCE Format   177
How to Develop a Selection OSCE   179
Evaluating the Utility of the Selection OSCE   182
Strengths and Limitations of the Selection OSCE   183
Summary   183
References   184

**Appendix 15.1   An Example of a Selection
                    OSCE Station**   185
Instructions to the Candidate   185
Instructions to the Simulated Friend   185
Instructions to the Examiner   186
List of Equipment   188

**Chapter 16   Frequently Asked Questions about
                the OSCE**   189
What is the Optimum Number of
   Stations in an OSCE?   189
What Should be the Length of Each Station?   189
Should there be Two Examiners per
   Station or One Examiner per Station?   190
Can We have an OSCE with Variable
   Durations of Stations?   190
Do We Need to have a Rest Station in an OSCE?   191
Do We Need Expert Examiners for an OSCE?   191
Can We Include Non-Physicians
   as OSCE Examiners?   191
Should the Patient Mark the OSCE Station?   192
Should the Examiners Provide Feedback
   to the Candidate during the OSCE?   192

Should the Examiners Ask Questions
of the Candidate during the OSCE?   192
Can We have Real Patients in an OSCE?   193
Can We Use Clinical Photographs in an OSCE?   193
Should there be Any "Killer" Stations in an OSCE?   193
Can We have Two OSCE Stations that
are Linked Together?   194
Which One of the Two Marking Methods,
Checklist or Rating, is Superior?   194
How Many Items Should a Checklist Contain?   195
How Can We Determine the Pass/Fail
Mark of the OSCE?   195
How Do We Maintain Examination Security
when there are Multiple Sessions?   195
How Should We Select a Venue for the OSCE?   196
How Can We Run an OSCE Over Two Days?   196
Can We Videotape OSCE Stations?   197
How Much Time do We Need to Prepare
for an OSCE?   197

Index   199
Authors' Biographies   203

1

THE BIRTH AND PROPAGATION OF THE OSCE

"Those who do not remember the past are condemned to repeat it."

George Santayana

In this opening chapter, our aim is to present a broad overview of the historical context of the birth of the OSCE, especially the factors that contributed to the development and propagation of the OSCE. We firmly believe that understanding the historical background is important for various reasons:

- It allows us to analyze the preceding events leading to the development of the OSCE.
- We develop a deeper understanding of the context of the OSCE in contemporary medical education and assessment.
- We learn from previous successes and mistakes, so that we can meaningfully implement the OSCE in our own settings.
- It prompts us to appreciate the enormous contributions of early doyens of medical education.

At the end of the chapter, we should be able to:

(i) Recognize how the shortcomings of traditional clinical examinations led to the birth of the OSCE.
(ii) Evaluate some of the seminal publications and events related to the development of the OSCE.
(iii) Compare and contrast early OSCE formats with contemporary OSCE formats.

The Birth

The development of the OSCE is rightly and widely credited to Professor Ronald McGregor Harden. In a seminal paper, published in the *British Medical Journal* in 1975, Harden *et al.* described a new approach to the assessment of clinical competence. However, even before the publication of this paper, there were considerable discussions in the medical literature highlighting the many shortfalls of traditional clinical examinations (Fleming *et al.*, 1974; Harden *et al.*, 1969; Wilson *et al.*, 1969). In traditional clinical examinations, there are typically one or two long cases where the candidate takes a history, performs a physical examination, reviews investigations, generates a differential diagnosis, and discusses the findings, interpretation, and general management options with the examiners. The long cases are supplemented with a few short cases, where the candidate's task is more defined with a focused history or physical examination followed by a brief discussion with the examiners.

The traditional clinical examinations have several drawbacks. Firstly, it is difficult to have certains types of real patients such as patients with shortness of breath or acute chest pain during the clinical examination. Secondly, the decision about a candidate's competency in clinical settings is based on a very limited number of encounters. Thirdly, the lack of clear instructions to the candidates and to the examiners renders the marking of candidates vulnerable to the examiners' moods, personal preferences, and prejudices.

Fourthly, the long cases, which typically use a patient from the ward or a previously known patient who has been called back from home, do not really represent the variety of patients a graduating doctor is expected to manage in real life. They are also heavily skewed towards in-patients. Finally, the logistical and practical difficulties of using real patients for the entire duration of the examination can be a daunting task and is ethically questionable.

Harden *et al.* (1975) summed up the above observations that traditional clinical examinations, with two examiners assessing the candidate's skills on only a few patients, are often "luck of the draw." The lack of clear instructions and prior discussions about the patient among the examiners also creates confusions regarding what should be tested and the expected level of competency required to pass the examination. In short, the crucial pass/fail decision generated during traditional clinical examinations is often arbitrary and depends on multiple confounding factors, including variability among the examiners, varying levels of complexity of patients, and the nature of illnesses. Simply speaking, such examinations are educationally, morally, and legally indefensible.

Harden was the Head of Division of Clinical Medical Education at the University of Dundee, UK (interview with Harden; Vimeo), when he and his colleagues wrote the groundbreaking paper on the OSCE in 1975. To counter some of the ills of the traditional clinical examination, Harden *et al.* (1975) proposed an "objective structured examination." Interestingly, the term "OSCE" did not appear in the original paper. The format of the clinical examination first proposed by Harden *et al.* was different from what we might be familiar with now. It had 16 stations (the number 16 was chosen because it was "convenient"). The duration at each station was 5 minutes. However, the stations included a mixture of clinical skills stations, observations/inspections of clinical materials, such as colored photographs, and written questions in the form of true/false multiple choice questions (MCQs). Thus, a typical configuration would look like this (Fig. 1.1).

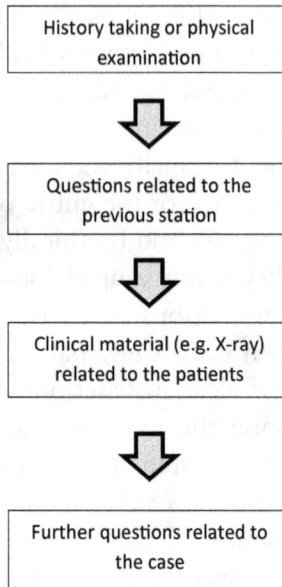

Fig. 1.1. Basic configuration of the early OSCE.

Each of these stations had clear instructions to the candidate, such as "Auscultate the precordium for evidence of valvular disease," after which the candidate would move onto another station, where they would answer questions relating to their findings from the previous station. The questions could be open-ended or multiple choice type, although, for convenience, true/false multiple choice-type questions were often used (Harden *et al.*, 1975). The examiners' checklist was rather simple in early examinations, with only "yes" and "no" options for each of the tasks performed. The checklist was later modified to allow a "qualified yes." The new format of objective structured examination was piloted with a limited number of volunteer students and examiners. It received an enthusiastic response from the students and somewhat lukewarm response from the examiners. Students viewed the format as fairer and less dependent on luck (interview with Harden; Vimeo) and supported its implementation.

We should also review another early development that took place in North America that preceded the publication of the landmark paper by Harden *et al.* in 1975. This had a profound effect on the OSCE format as we practice now. Howard Barrows was an Assistant Professor of Neurology and Stephen Abrahamson was the Director of Research in Medical Education at the University of Southern California, School of Medicine, Los Angeles, CA, USA. They experimented with "programmed patients" as a way of appraising students' performance in clinical neurology (Barrows and Abrahamson, 1964). They argued, among others, that patients are inherently prone to presenting their findings variably to the students and that an ideal patient that suits the needs of the examination is often hard to come by.

Therefore, they suggested training "programmed patients," which involved "simulation of disease by a normal person who is trained to assume and present, on examination, the history and neurological findings of an actual patient in the manner of an actual patient" (Barrows and Abrahamson, 1964). Programmed patients, as we now know, have been expanded to include both "standardized patients" and "simulated patients." Barrows and Abrahamson used programmed patients to "obtain appraisal of the student's clinical performance" — a feat that might seem revolutionary to some, even four decades later. Further down the road, simulation and mannequins would become an integral part of the repository of clinical materials that can be tested during a clinical examination.

Programmed patients brought greater standardization to the clinical presentation of patients and reduced the variability that is inherent with the use of real patients. Harden *et al.* merged two emerging assessment techniques of that age: Programmed patients for standardization and multi-station examination by multiple examiners working independently in order to assess several domains at the same time (Hodges, 2003). Although these two ideas, taken separately, were neither novel nor revolutionary, marrying them

> 👆 **Good to Know**
>
> - Standardized patients: real patients or actors portraying findings in a standardized manner
> - Simulated patients: trained actors acting as patients
> - Simulation: enacting a clinical scenario
> - Simulator: mechanical devises, mannequins with or without intelligent features

together in a systematic manner to test clinical competency was unique (Hodges, 2003).

OSCE as a Global Phenomenon

Acceptance of the OSCE was further bolstered by continuous research and refinements, not only regarding the OSCE, but also regarding the nature of clinical competencies, appreciation of holistic roles of physicians, and psychometrics of assessment in medical education (Khan *et al.*, 2013). Some of the crucial evidence related to the OSCE, as a method of student assessment, will be discussed in the subsequent chapters.

In the last two decades, anecdotal observations and professional experience support the notion that the pace of adoption of the OSCE as a preferred method of student assessment has accelerated considerably across the globe, from undergraduate to postgraduate settings. Many professional bodies and national licensing examinations have endorsed and adopted the OSCE or its variations as a standard clinical assessment across the spectrum of physician training. For example, after years of reliance on knowledge assessment through MCQs, most medical schools in the USA now use the OSCE or similar examinations for clinical assessment (Turner and Dankoski, 2008). National licensing authorities, including the National Board of Medical Examiners, USA

(USMLE 2 CS), the Medical Council of Canada (Medical Council of Canada Qualifying Examination Part II), the General Medical Council, UK (PLAB Part 2), among others, are now regularly using the OSCE or its variants in high-stakes summative decision-making.

Key milestones

- 1979: Publication of *"Assessment of Clinical Competence Using an Objective Structured Clinical Examination (OSCE)"* as an Association for the Study of Medical Education (ASME) Guide by Harden and Gleeson
- 1985: 1st Ottawa Conference on Assessment of Clinical Competency brought the idea of the OSCE to North America
- 1998: Australian Medical Council conducted an OSCE for the first time for licensing foreign medical graduates to practice in Australia
- 1998: Education Commission for Foreign Medical Graduates, USA (ECFMG) conducted large-scale OSCEs in the USA for the first time
- 2000: Publication of ACGME Toolbox of Assessment Methods (2000) endorsed the OSCE as the one of the preferred methods of assessment of clinical competency

Summary

The OSCE did not originate in a vacuum. Much impetus towards the development of the OSCE came from the recognition of many serious flaws associated with unstructured, unstandardized traditional clinical examinations, where the decision often depended on a sole examiner (or a few examiners) examining one or few aspects of clinical competency. The OSCE reduced bias, provided clearer instruction to the examiners and candidates, and changed the perception that "clinical examination is often a game of luck."

References

Barrows HS, Abrahamson S. (1964) The programmed patient: A technique for appraising students' performance in clinical neurology. *J Med Educ* **39**: 802–804.

Fleming PR, Manderson WG, Matthews MB, Sanderson PH, Stokes JF. (1974) Evolution of an examination: M.R.C.P. (U.K.). *Br Med J* **13**; 2(5910): 99–102.

Harden RM, Gleeson FA. (1979) Assessment of clinical competence using an objective structured clinical examination (OSCE). Medical Education Booklet No. 8. *Med Educ* **13**(1): 41–54.

Harden RM, Stevenson M, Downie WW, Wilson GM. (1975) Assessment of clinical competence using objective structured examination. *Br Med J* **1**(5955): 447–451.

Hodges B. (2003) OSCE! Variations on a theme by Harden. *Med Educ* **37**(12): 1134–1140.

Interview with Professor Ronald Harden about the OSCE. Centre for Medical Education Dundee. Website: http://vimeo.com/67224904 (Accessed on 20 February 2014).

Khan KZ, Ramachandran S, Gaunt K, Pushkar P. (2013) The Objective Structured Clinical Examination (OSCE): AMEE Guide No. 81. Part I: A historical and theoretical perspective. *Med Teach* **35**: e1437–e1446.

Shumway JM, Harden RM. (2003) AMEE Guide No. 25: The assessment of learning outcomes for the competent and reflective physicians. *Med Teach* **25**(6): 569–584.

Toolbox of Assessment Methods. ACGME Outcomes Project. (2000) Accreditation Council for Graduate Medical Education (ACGME) and American Board of Medical Specialities (ABMS). Version 1.1. Available at: [http://www.chd.ubc.ca/files/file/instructor-resources/Evaluation toolbox.pdf] (Accessed on 28 February 2014).

Wilson GM, Lever R, Harden RM. Robertson JIS, Macritchie J. (1969) Examination of clinical examiners. *The Lancet* **293**(7584): 37–40.

2

THE OSCE IN THE CONTEXT OF A HOLISTIC ASSESSMENT

"The OSCE) is in essence a clinical or practical examination in which aspects of clinical competencies are sampled to determine students' clinical skills and abilities related to their competence to practise medicine."

Shumway and Harden (2003)

The OSCE is one of several methods of assessment required to obtain a holistic profile of a candidate. Therefore, it is imperative that we critically examine how the OSCE fits into the overall assessment plan. This chapter provides a broad overview of the OSCE by discussing what an OSCE is, how an OSCE can be used along with other methods of assessment, how an OSCE would be typically configured, and why the OSCE has won special attention and preference among medical teachers as a way of assessing clinical competence.

At the end of the chapter, we should be able to:

(i) Recognize the place of the OSCE in the context of clinical assessment.

(ii) Discuss the configuration of a typical OSCE.

(iii) Analyze why the OSCE is considered to be a useful form of clinical assessment at the "Shows how" level of the Miller's pyramid.

(iv) Compare and contrast the OSCE with other forms of clinical assessment, such as the short cases and the mini-clinical evaluation exercise (mini-CEX).

(v) Distinguish the real OSCE from the OSCE pretenders.

How Does the OSCE Fit into Overall Assessment?

The OSCE is a form of assessment that assesses clinical competencies such as history taking, physical examination, communication skills, ethics, attitudes, and professionalism under examination conditions; i.e. in simulated situations (Harden *et al.*, 1975; Harden, 1988; Newble, 2004). Since these competencies are being tested under examination conditions, as opposed to real-life or clinical practice situations, the OSCE is considered to assess the candidate at the "Shows how" level in the classification of medical assessment by Miller (1990); i.e. Miller's pyramid (Fig. 2.1).

If we examine Fig. 2.1, it is clearly apparent that the OSCE needs to be supplemented by other methods of assessment in order to obtain a holistic profile about the candidate. Typically, cognition or knowledge is assessed by different forms of written or computer-based assessment, such as MCQs, short answer questions, or modified essay questions. Behavior, broadly defined as what we can do and carry out, is assessed through task-based activities. These task-based activities can be assessed in examination situations (i.e. *in vitro*) or in real-life situations (i.e. *in vivo*).

Typically, the OSCE is utilized for the assessment of clinical skills in examination settings, because an examination set-up provides

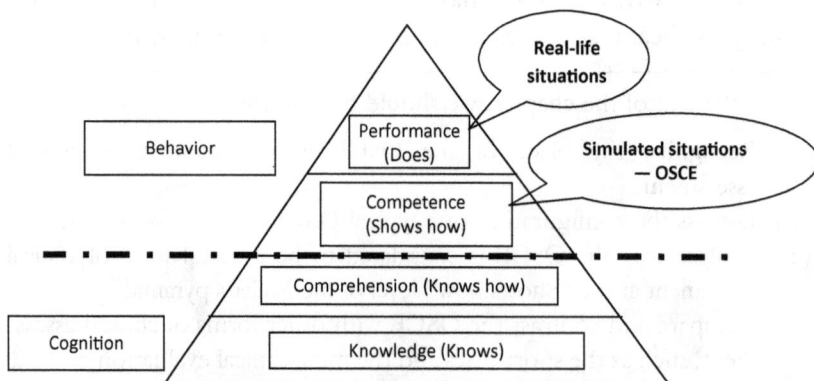

Fig. 2.1.   Miller's pyramid of assessment (Miller, 1990).

the requisite structure, convenience, and control to enforce the necessary rigor for making a critical decision such as graduating a doctor. In an OSCE, just like other examination situations, the candidate, under the observation of an examiner, may pretend to carry out a given task in a perfect manner. Of course, that does not guarantee whether he/she will really carry out the task even when he/she is unobserved.

As we move up the pyramid, task-based activities can be tested in real-life situations or *in vivo* as well. Such assessments take place with real patients in an actual clinical environment, such as wards, emergency rooms, clinics, or operating theatres. The assessment instruments used for this purpose include mini-CEX and direct observation of procedural skills (DOPS), among others. Some, however, could argue that these assessments may not exactly capture the real-life performance of the candidate, since a candidate may only pretend to carry out a task in a perfect manner when observed by an examiner (i.e. during the examination).

If we are really interested in finding out whether a practitioner is performing his/her tasks even when unobserved, we have to collect data from the real-life practice environment in an unobtrusive manner; i.e. through feedback from patients, having an unannounced trained patient in the clinic, or more commonly through anonymous collection of feedback from a range of peers or other healthcare professionals and patients. The latter is also called multisource feedback. However, despite the authenticity and attractiveness of such direct methods, patients and other healthcare professionals may not have the requisite knowledge to judge many major components of clinical skills, such as application of knowledge, clinical reasoning, and clinical judgments. In addition, there are inherent logistical difficulties in organizing a robust system for collecting data in the clinical setting and isolating performance of the physician from other unrelated factors that affect the ratings (Singh & Norcini, 2013).

As can be seen in the foregoing discussion, the behaviors assessed at "Shows how" and "Does" levels are fundamentally different. Hence, some have developed a nomenclature that assigns the term "competence" to indicate the "Shows how" level and the term "performance" to indicate the "Does" level (Rethans *et al.*, 2002). Since such nomenclature is not adopted worldwide, and for the sake of simplicity, we have used these two terms interchangeably in this book.

Thus, any single method is insufficient to obtain a holistic profile of a candidate's competence. As such, there has to be a rational and balanced representation of various methods in order to obtain a comprehensive profile of a candidate. The OSCE is not an exception to this rule. The OSCE is efficient in capturing certain aspects of a candidate's competence (i.e. clinical skills in examination settings), whereas it is less efficient in assessing knowledge or performance at the workplace.

Basic Configuration of an OSCE

The OSCE assesses clinical competencies using brief, discrete tasks that reflect a healthcare professional's day-to-day activities, such as taking a history of the presenting complaint, examining the cardiovascular system, breaking bad news, and giving health advice on nutrition, among others. Such tasks, almost as a rule, represent patient encounters or clinically related hands-on activities.

An OSCE task should:

➢ Focus on clinically important aspects of competence
➢ Be based on hands-on activities; i.e. assessment of pure knowledge should not be considered to be an OSCE task
➢ Assess competencies that cannot be tested in a written assessment

In an OSCE, each task is organized within a standalone unit of assessment called the "station." An OSCE contains several stations running in parallel within an OSCE circuit. Figure 2.2 illustrates such an OSCE circuit.

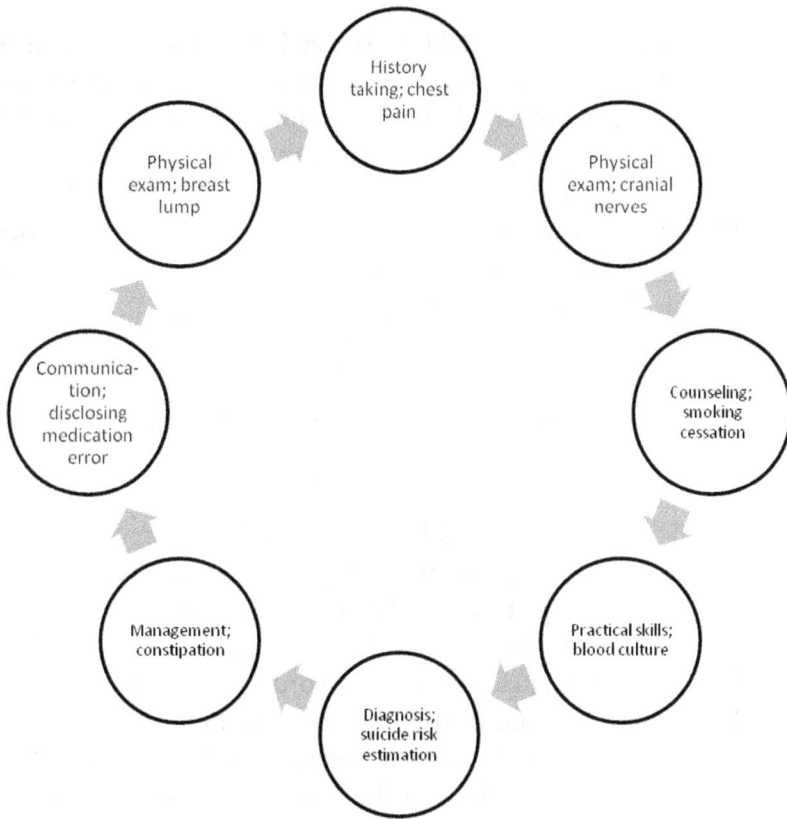

Fig. 2.2. Basic configuration of an OSCE. (Note the range of skill sets tested. Ideally, the number of stations should be more. Only the main competence tested in each station has been mentioned.)

Typically, all stations have the same time duration. Hence, a candidate can start the OSCE from any point (i.e. any station) within the circuit and move station by station until the completion of all the stations. Thus, the number of candidates that can take the OSCE at a given time (i.e. within a single run of an OSCE circuit) is determined by the number of stations within the circuit. If the number of candidates is more than the number of stations, for all candidates to complete the OSCE, either the same circuit has to be repeated several times or several parallel circuits need to be set up.

> The special appeal of the OSCE format is that the multitude of tasks that an OSCE assesses is not only based on a range of patients representing different conditions, but also each task is assessed independently by a different examiner. Therefore, the OSCE manages to sample not only the clinical materials (i.e. patients with different clinical conditions) and the competencies being assessed (e.g. physical examination, communication skills, and history taking), but also the examiners.

It is noteworthy that these specific, brief and discrete tasks have two distinct features.

(i) Specificity: A task in an OSCE station is defined in terms of its specificity, providing the exact activity that candidates need to carry out, such that the candidates' actions related to a given task should only vary due to the different ability levels of the different candidates. In other words, candidates' actions should not vary due to the vagueness of the prescribed tasks where different candidates may interpret that same task differently or due to variations in the conditions (e.g. variations in the presentation of the patients) under which each candidate carries out the task.

(ii) Brevity (i.e. being a sample of a more holistic or larger activity): A given OSCE task (i.e. an OSCE station) is not a "comprehensive" representation of an activity that a healthcare professional carries out. For example, a task in an OSCE, such as examination of the cardiovascular system, is only a sample (or a subcomponent) of the more holistic task of a physical examination that a healthcare professional typically carries out.

The above two features (i.e. specificity and brevity) can, however, also be viewed as a relative disadvantage, in that specific and brief tasks do not lend themselves to assessing the curriculum in its entirety (i.e. all of the tasks in which a candidate should be assessed). A comprehensive OSCE, involving many stations, overcomes these disadvantages by assessing multiple brief of tasks.

Why is an OSCE Preferable Over Traditional Clinical Examinations?

Traditionally, in health professional examination, history taking and physical examination skills were assessed using long cases and short cases. These assessments, however, had several shortcomings:

(i) Subjective assessment: In the classical long cases and short cases, the examiners did not use a standardized marking scheme, such as a rating scale or a checklist. Hence, different examiners employed different criteria to judge a candidate's competence.

(ii) Unstructured nature of assessment: No two candidates were assessed on the same clinical material, as different candidates encountered different patients. Similarly, different candidates may have ended up being assessed by different examiner panels. Hence, the scores of two candidates were virtually incomparable.

(iii) Inability to assess the ability to carry out medical procedures: The long cases and short cases only assessed history taking and physical examination skills. They did not assess medical procedures such as intravenous cannulation, cardiopulmonary resuscitation, or lumbar puncture, among others.

(iv) Inability to sample the curriculum adequately: The classical long case took about 45–60 min to assess a candidate based on a single patient (Norcini, 2002; Norman, 2002), while the number of short cases were typically confined to four or five patients, each lasting 5–10 minutes. This limited the ability of the examination to test a range of clinical conditions and tasks necessary for making an informed decision on a candidate's ability (Ponnamperuma *et al.*, 2009).

Shortfalls of traditional clinical examinations:

- Only a limited skill set could be tested in the examination
- Decisions about a candidate's competency were based on limited encounters
- No clear-cut instruction were given to the candidates, the examiners, or the patients
- There may have been a lack of consistency between the examiners; i.e. marking criteria of examiners may have varied widely
- Patients varied across candidates
- Recruiting real patients for the examination was logistically difficult
- Exposing real patients repeatedly as test materials was ethically debatable

The OSCE was proposed to mitigate the above deficiencies. How does the OSCE overcome the above deficiencies? Well, the answer is within the four words of the OSCE:

(i) Objective: The OSCE uses a checklist or rating scale that specifically requests the examiner to look for particular aspects related to a candidate's ability when a candidate carries out a task. Not only does it force the examiner to observe these specific abilities, but the OSCE also requires the examiners to pass a judgment about the candidate's ability on these aspects using specific marking criteria.

(ii) Structured: All candidates are assessed using the same or similar examination materials. They are also assessed by the same or similarly trained examiners who use the same assessment criteria.

(iii) Clinical: The OSCE has the capacity to assess not only the history taking and physical examination of a candidate, but is also capable of accommodating much broader domains of a physician's competencies, such as medical procedures. In addition, it can be used to assess a candidate's skills and attributes that are auxiliary to history taking, physical examination, and medical procedures, such as communication skills, professionalism, ethics, and attitudes.

(iv) Examination: Due to the short duration that a given task lasts, the OSCE is an "examination" in the true sense of the word, as it is intrinsically capable of accommodating a relatively large number of clinical encounters; e.g. clinical conditions and procedures.

The ability of the OSCE to assess multiple domains of physician competency deserves further exploration. Studies in cognitive psychology and the nature of expertise have highlighted the fact that there is a high degree of context and case specificity (Eva, 2003; Regehr & Norman, 1996) in clinical practice. Simply speaking, a physician's ability to deal with clinical problems tends to be context and case specific. Physicians do not possess generic problem-solving skills. For example, a physician may be very good at diagnosing asthma but poor at diagnosing rheumatoid arthritis. Therefore, an examination that assesses a candidate's ability to diagnose one specific condition is not rigorous enough to conclude whether the same candidate would be equally good at diagnosing or managing another condition. To overcome the problem of case and context specificity, we need to assess candidates in a range of clinical conditions. The OSCE provides us with an opportunity to assess a candidate based on multiple clinical conditions, and hence it counters the context and case specificity that are typically present with long or short cases.

Advantages of the OSCE

- The OSCE tests a range of clinical competencies and conditions that are germane to clinical medicine, including medical emergencies and psychiatric diseases, which are seldom tested in traditional clinical examinations;
- The OSCE allows objective and more uniform assessments of these competencies through uniform instructions and marking schemes;
- The decision about the candidate's ability is based on a panel of examiners rather than a single examiner;
- The OSCE collects data about the candidate's competencies during the examination that can be used for individual or cohort feedback or improvement of the curriculum;

- The OSCE minimizes the use of real patients in the examination, thereby ensuring patient comfort, safety, and confidentiality.

Disadvantages of the OSCE

- Skills are tested in the OSCE in brief encounters rather than as a whole; this may discourage students to evaluate a patient holistically;
- Too much standardization and objectivity may promote ritualistic and stereotypical behaviors; students may go through the process of performing the tasks without thinking critically;
- The OSCE is resource intensive; it requires significant organizational ability to implement an examination flawlessly.

In the following chapters, we will learn how we can minimize the disadvantages of the OSCE through careful planning and implementation.

OSCE, Short Cases, and the Mini-CEX

Short cases and the mini-CEX are two popular examination methods that bear some similarities with the OSCE. All three methods depend on multiple patient encounters or clinical cases in order to assess candidates. Assessment is based on direct observation of the candidate. All three also focus on clinical skills that cannot be tested in paper-and-pencil examinations. The short cases and the OSCE take place in examination situations and assess a candidate at the "Shows how" level of Miller's pyramid (Table 2.1). By contrast, the mini-CEX takes place with real patients within more authentic clinical settings and assesses candidate at the "Does" level of Miller's pyramid (Table 2.2).

Table 2.1. A Comparison Between the Short Cases and the OSCE Examination Methods

Features	Short Cases	OSCE	OSCE-related Impact on Examination
Number of patients/ clinical cases	Generally up to four	Generally 12–16	Greater content validity and reliability
Focus	Mostly on physical examination skills	Comprehensive range of clinical skills	Greater validity
Examiners	One examiner may be responsible for examining all candidates	Independent examiners for each station	Collective decision of all examiners
Patients	Real patients	Mixture of standardized patients, simulated patients, and mannequins	Broader range of competencies (e.g. patient safety) can be assessed
Marking template	Generic; applicable to all cases	Station or case specific	Greater objectivity

OSCE Pretenders or Imitation OSCEs

Experience suggests that many institutions conduct OSCEs that are in gross violation of the basic educational principles underpinning good assessment. We should categorically object to these pretenders as they are detrimental to students' learning and ultimately to patient wellbeing. Examples include:

- A multi-station examination where students rotate through different stations just like a real OSCE. However, tasks are limited to testing of knowledge in the form of interpretation of short

Table 2.2.   Differences between the OSCE and the Mini-CEX

Features	OSCE	Mini-CEX
Level of assessment	"Shows how" level in Miller's pyramid	"Does" level in Miller's pyramid
Set-up	Examination settings	Clinical settings; e.g. in-patients, out-patients, and emergency rooms
Variables (patients, examiners, and difficulty levels)	More controlled	Less controlled
Number of patients/clinical cases	12–16 for good range of content coverage	6–8 per year for good coverage
Standardization	More	Less
Marking template	Specific for individual station	Generic

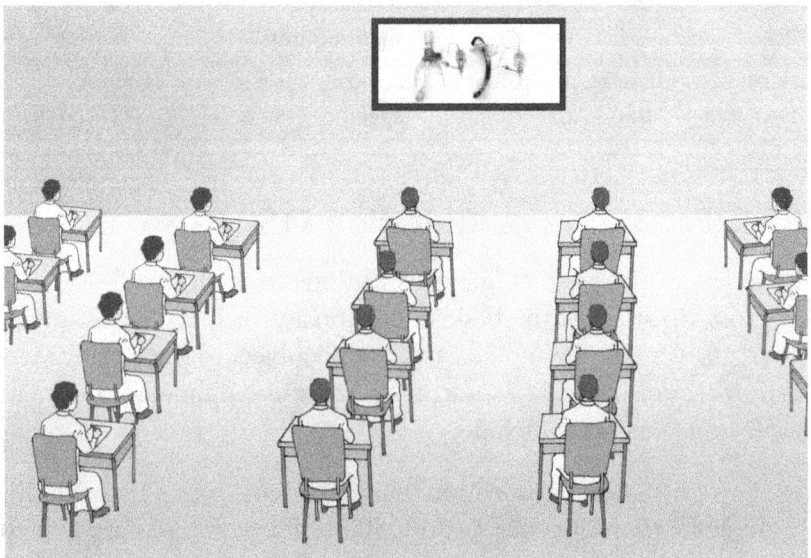

Fig. 2.3.   Students being examined in an examination room with projected material as the content of the so-called stations. There is no clinical task — this is not an OSCE!

answer questions, clinical images, X-rays, laboratory findings, and tissue specimens, etc. There are no real clinical tasks involved, such as history taking or clinical examination.

- Students sit down in an examination room. Examiners project clinical photographs and students write answers in the paper-and-pencil format (Fig. 2.3).
- In an examination, students are asked to perform clinical skills. Examiners rate the students based on a specific checklist. However, there are only one or two stations, which limits the content validity of the examination.

Summary

The OSCE is a form of clinical assessment that assesses competencies such as history taking, physical examination, and communication skills, among others, under simulated (i.e. examination) conditions using the day-to-day activities of a healthcare professional. These activities, which may represent only a part (e.g. auscultating the precordium) of a more comprehensive activity (e.g. history taking and physical examination, which includes the auscultation of the precordium), are organized into stations as specific and brief tasks. Several such stations arranged within a sequential circuit form the entire OSCE. The psychometric appeal of the OSCE is that it is an examination format that assesses the "Shows how" level of Miller's pyramid by sampling through a multitude of patients, disease conditions, and examiners. Such an assessment format is more objective, structured, and clinical in its orientation.

References

Eva KW. (2003) On the generality of specificity. *Med Educ* **37**(7): 587–588.

Harden RM, Stevenson M, Downie WW, Wilson GM. (1975) Assessment of clinical competence using objective structured examination. *Br Med J* **1**(5955): 447–451.

Harden RM. (1988) What is an OSCE? *Med Teach* **10**(1): 19–23.

Miller G. (1990) The assessment of clinical skills/competence/performance. *Acad Med* **65**(Suppl.): S63–S67.

Newble D. (2004) Techniques of measuring clinical competence: Objective structured clinical examination. *Med Educ* **38**(2): 199–203.

Norcini JJ, Blank LL, Duffy FD, Fortna G. (2003) The mini-CEX: A method for assessing clinical skills. *Ann Intern Med* **138**(6): 476–481.

Norcini JJ. (2002) The death of the long case? *Br Med J* **324**(7334): 408–409.

Norman G. (2002) The long case versus objective structured clinical examination. *Br Med J* **324**(7340): 748–749.

Ponnamperuma GG, Karunathilake IM, McAleer S, Davis MH. (2009) The long case and its modifications: A literature review. *Med Educ* **43**(10): 936–941.

Regehr G, Norman GR. (1996) Issues in cognitive psychology: Implications for professional education. *Acad Med* **71**(9): 988–1001.

Rethans J-J, Norcini JJ, Barón-Maldonado M, Blackmore D, Jolly BC, LaDuca T, Lew S, Page GG, Southgate LH. (2002) The relationship between competence and performance: Implications for assessing practice performance. *Med Educ* **36**(10): 901–909.

Shumway JM, Harden RM. (2003) AMEE Guide No. 25: The assessment of learning outcomes for the competent and reflective physician. *Med Teach* **25**: 569–584.

Singh T, Norcini JJ. (2013) Workplace-based assessment. In: McGaghie WC (ed.), *International Best Practices for Evaluation in the Health Professions*, Radcliffe Publishing, UK, pp. 257–280.

3

VALUE OF THE OSCE
AS AN ASSESSMENT TOOL

In the previous two chapters, we discussed the birth and the propagation of the OSCE, and how the OSCE fits into the overall assessment plan. In this chapter, we shall delve deeper into understanding the value of the OSCE as an assessment tool.

Overall value or utility of an assessment method depends on multiple factors. van der Vleuten (1996) neatly summarized five important elements that impact the value or utility of an assessment method: validity, reliability, educational impact, acceptability, and cost. Of these five, validity and reliability are two psychometric properties, while educational impact, acceptability, and cost are non-psychometric factors. We shall use van der Vleuten's utility criteria with minor modifications in order to evaluate how we can employ the different psychometric and non-psychometric measures to improve the overall value of the OSCE.

At the end of this chapter, we should be able to:

(i) Explain the factors influencing the value of the OSCE as an assessment method.
(ii) Recognize the relationship between validity and reliability.
(iii) Propose practical measures to enhance the value of the OSCE.
(iv) Discuss a sampling strategy that influences the validity and reliability of an OSCE.

☝ **Good to Know**

- Validity: The ability of a test to measure what it intends to measure
- Reliability: The consistency of test scores across examiners, different testing conditions, and multiple time frames; i.e. the underlying principle that ensures such consistency of scores aims towards minimization of the variability of test scores, except that which is due to the variability of candidates' ability
- Educational impact: The negative and positive influence of the examination on education in general and examinees in particular; i.e. the ability of an examination to drive the candidates towards meaningful learning
- Acceptability: How well the examination is perceived by different stakeholders, such as examinees, examiners, regulatory bodies, and the public
- Practicality: The feasibility and cost–benefit of conducting the examination

Validity

The validity of a test refers to the degree to which a test measures what it intends to measure (Barman, 2005; Downing, 2003). Validity is the single most important factor to consider in test construction (Newble, 1992). If the validity is compromised, the entire test becomes useless. Validity, unlike reliability, depends to an extent on experts' interpretations, rather than solely on statistical analysis.

There are many types of validity; e.g. content validity, concurrent validity, predictive validity, and construct validity. Although all of these types of validity are important, it is the content validity that one can definitively determine before administering a test. All other types of validity can only be calculated after administering the test; i.e. once the test scores are available. Hence, in this section, we only consider how we can ensure the content validity of an OSCE.

Content validity of an OSCE primarily depends on the extent to which the entire OSCE contains a representative sample of clinical competencies that the examinees are expected to achieve at the end of the course, both in terms of learning outcomes and curricular contents (Amin, Chong, & Khoo, 2006; Barman, 2005). Of course, this does not mean that the OSCE should have a representative sample from all domains and competencies to be tested. Other examination methods, such as written and work-based assessment methods, in conjunction with the OSCE, would provide a more comprehensive profile of competencies of the candidate. Therefore, the OSCE must be combined with other methods of assessment.

The most efficient way to achieve a representative sample of the curriculum is through a blueprint or a table of specification. A blueprint would ensure that important competencies are tested and that there is a rational representation of the content and learning outcomes in the examination. A detailed discussion on methods of improving the validity of the OSCE through blueprinting is presented in Chapter 4.

☝ **Good to Know**

Threat to validity: An Examination Committee of a given school was tasked to develop an OSCE for its final-year medical students. The purpose of the OSCE was to determine graduating medical students' abilities on a broad range of competencies that are germane to the practice of medicine. The Examination Committee had three members from medicine, surgery, and pediatrics. After several meetings, the Committee came up with eight stations. The stations were:

(i) Examination of the cardiovascular system of a patient with aortic regurgitation (discipline: Internal medicine; skills tested: Physical examination and diagnosis; content: Cardiovascular system)
(ii) Examination of the lower limbs of a patient with peripheral vascular diseases (discipline: Surgery; skills tested: Physical examination and diagnosis; content: Cardiovascular system)
(iii) History taking from a patient with chronic breathlessness (discipline: Internal medicine; skills tested: History taking and diagnosis; content: Respiratory system)

(Continued)

☞ **Good to Know** *(Continued)*

(iv) Demonstration of inhaler use (discipline: Pediatrics; skills tested: Counseling; content: Respiratory system)

(v) Taking consent for a lumber puncture (discipline: Pediatrics; skills tested: Counseling; content: Nervous system)

(vi) Examination of the gait of a patient with stroke (discipline: Internal medicine; skills tested: Physical examination and diagnosis; content: Nervous system)

(vii) Examination of the abdomen in a patient with jaundice (discipline: Surgery; skill tested: Physical examination and diagnosis; content: Gastrointestinal system)

(viii) Examination of an inguinal lump (discipline: Surgery; skill tested: Physical examination and diagnosis; content: Gastrointestinal system)

If we examine this list carefully, we can deduce that although the stations are important and relevant to the practice of medicine, there are significant overlaps as well as under-representation of certain disciplines, skills, and content areas. For example, physical examination skills are overemphasized, but there are no clinical problems related to acute medicine, mental health, and female health issues. The selection of stations and accompanying clinical material was based on convenience and their familiarity to the examiners. This threatens the validity of the examination.

Top three tips for improving the content validity of the OSCE:

- Assess all of the possible clinical competencies that an OSCE could assess;
- Sample the content areas as widely as possible;
- Maintain the right balance between competencies and content areas; i.e. ensure that the competencies and content areas are represented in adequate numbers and proportions, so that the important competencies and content areas are assessed proportionately more than the not-so-important content areas.

Reliability

Reliability refers to the reproducibility of the test scores over different time-frames, under different testing conditions, and between examiners, patients, etc. (Newble & Swanson, 1988). Reliability is often expressed in quantitative or statistical terms. For example, the type of reliability known as "inter-rater reliability" refers to the consistency of the markings between two (or more) examiners who are examining the same candidate at the same time using the same patients.

The key underlying principle that ensures the reproducibility of test scores is the minimization of the error associated with any test. This ensures that, as much as possible, the scores attributed to candidates reflect their ability, rather than other irrelevant factors, such as examiner biases or variable interpretations of the task that is undertaken by the candidates.

One of the most important factors that determine the reliability of an OSCE is the number of stations. Too few a number of stations in an OSCE would compromise its reliability, whereas increasing the number of stations would improve reliability.

Other factors that negatively influence the reliability of an OSCE include:

(i) Poorly trained standardized patients;
(ii) A poorly designed marking template;
(iii) An inadequate station duration;
(iv) Vague instructions to the examiners, candidates, and patients.

Self-learning Exercise

How do the factors mentioned above affect the reliability of the OSCE?

(Answers are at the end of the chapter.)

Top three tips for improving the reliability of the OSCE:

- Increase the number of stations by maximally distributing the available number of examiners; i.e. this implies employing one examiner per station as opposed to two examiners per station;
- Conduct thorough examiner briefings on expected competencies and the scoring template;
- Carefully check through the marking template to reduce inconsistencies and vagueness.

Diagonal Sampling Strategy to Improve Validity and Reliability

You might have noticed that both the validity and the reliability of the examination depend on the number of stations or competencies/content areas tested in the examination. However, increasing the number of stations also means requiring more examiners, more patients, and generally higher resource utilization. Let us have a critical look at how we can increase the number of stations to improve the validity and reliability without necessarily increasing the resources.

Let us think of two hypothetical scenarios involving a clinical examination.

In Scenario A (Table 3.1), there is one examiner. The examiner is assigned to examine candidates using five different patients (jaundice, diabetes, stroke, asthma, and headache). The examiner moves from one patient to the next along with the candidate. The examiner spends 8 minutes with each case. Therefore, the total examiner's time for a given candidate is 40 person-minutes (8 minutes × 5 cases).

In Scenario B, five examiners are assigned to examine a given candidate on a particular patient with jaundice. All five examiners are required to observe the candidate simultaneously and make independent decisions about the candidate's competency in the given station. Like Scenario A, examiners are required to spend 8 minutes

Table 3.1. Scenario A — One Examiner Assessing Candidates on Five Different Cases

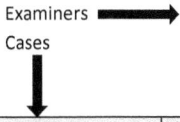

Examiners ➡

Cases ⬇

	Examiner 1				
Jaundice: Clinical examination	X				
Diabetes: Counseling	X				
Stroke: Rehabilitation	X				
Asthma: Use of inhaler	X				
Headache: History	X				

Table 3.2. Scenario B — Five Examiners Assessing a Candidate on a Single Case

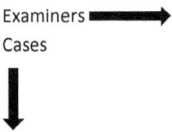

Examiners ➡

Cases ⬇

	Examiner 1	Examiner 2	Examiner 3	Examiner 4	Examiner 5
Jaundice: Clinical examination	X	X	X	X	X

with the candidate. Therefore, the total examiners' time per candidate is also 40 person-minutes (8 minutes × 5 examiners). Table 3.2 schematically represents the set-up of this examination.

Let us consider the relative advantages and disadvantages of these two scenarios. Scenario A's main advantage is that it has a greater range of competencies tested in the examination. The candidate has the opportunity to be tested on five different scenarios with different tasks. Scenario A provides much better sampling of contents when compared to Scenario B, in which the candidate is tested on only one case. In other words, Scenario A has much better content validity than Scenario B. However, in Scenario A, the decisions are made by one examiner, and therefore, such decisions are inherently prone to the bias of that given examiner.

In Scenario B, the candidate is tested on only one case by five different examiners. Scenario B does not have enough representativeness of the content, which reduces its content validity. However, Scenario B has less chance of examiner bias than Scenario A. Even if there is an outlier among the five examiners (i.e. an overtly lenient or a very strict examiner), this particular examiner's influence would be mitigated by the four other examiners.

Table 3.3 summarizes the findings of the two scenarios.

Table 3.3.   The Trade-off Effect of Validity and Reliability in Scenario A and Scenario B

	Validity	Reliability
Scenario A	High	Low
Scenario B	Low	High

Since both scenarios utilize the same examiners' time and have relative merits and disadvantages, the question is whether we can merge the good features of these two scenarios and devise a better test design that would increase validity and reliability without significantly increasing the required resources. Here is a diagonal sampling strategy (Table 3.4) that takes into account the good features from both scenarios. This diagonal sampling strategy with multiple independent examiners is an essential attribute of the design of an examination and a fundamental principle governing the OSCE.

Educational Impact

Any assessment can potentially impact education either positively or negatively. The OSCE can modulate the behavior of the examinees

Table 3.4. Diagonal Sampling Strategy for Increasing an Examination's Validity and Reliability

	Examiner 1	Examiner 2	Examiner 3	Examiner 4	Examiner 5
Jaundice: Clinical examination	X				
Diabetes: Counseling		X			
Stroke: Rehabilitation			X		
Asthma: Use of inhaler				X	
Headache: History					X

and examiners and can inform curriculum implementers of the potential weaknesses and strengths of the program. However, if improperly used and implemented, the OSCE can have a potentially negative impact on education as well.

Let us consider an example how an OSCE can positively affect learning and behavior. A given institute faced the problem of insulin overdosing by its junior doctors. On several occasions, the doctors either prescribed incorrectly or gave overdoses of insulin to the patients, resulting in severe consequences. An OSCE station was designed where the examinees' tasks were to review the dose of insulin, draw the right amount of insulin with the right syringe, check that the correct amount of insulin was drawn, and administer the insulin properly to a mannequin. During the post-examination review, it was revealed that a substantial number of examinee doctors failed at this particular station. Further analysis revealed two recurring critical mistakes for failure: (a) Examinees using the wrong syringes; and (b) examinees failing to countercheck the dose with the accompanying nurse. During the post-examination briefing, examinee doctors complained that they did not have sufficient opportunity to learn these skills during their training. The institute developed and offered a short course on medication safety to all junior doctors that emphasized how to select the correct syringe and the importance of counterchecking the dose with the nurse before administering insulin to patients. In subsequent years, similar OSCE stations were included. Almost all the examinees performed the steps correctly and administered the right amount of insulin. The institute noted a declining number of insulin overdoses in the ensuing years.

Let us consider another example, but this time considering how an OSCE can have a negative impact on education. In a particular OSCE station, candidates were given 5 minutes to take a complete history from a patient with chronic pain. The marking was based on a checklist that captured what the examinee was supposed to do. Examinees' scores depended on completing the list efficiently within the given period of time. During the OSCE, examinees were forced to go through as many of the checklist items as possible within the allocated time. In the process, the examinees often interrupted the patient, preventing them from telling their complete story. After the examination was over, the details regarding the OSCE were spread to other students who started preparing in a similar manner for their upcoming OSCE.

Top three tips for improving the educational impact of the OSCE:

- In the OSCE, include stations focusing on important content areas and competencies of practical relevance that you want the candidates to master, using an assessment blueprint.
- Include an itemized marking template, in addition to the global marking for each station, in order to identify recurring deficiencies in the candidate.
- Modify the stations for the future, if necessary, by carefully evaluating qualitative and quantitative data about student performance and feedback from examiners, students, and other stakeholders during the post-examination review.

The students' behavior was modulated adversely by this OSCE. Students were forced to learn to take histories in a hurried, unkind, non-explorative manner.

Acceptability

The acceptability of the OSCE to the students, faculty, administrators, and public is important for the long-term sustainability of the examination. Acceptability of the examination promotes credibility of the graduating doctors. It depends on how the OSCE is perceived by the various stakeholders. Some refer to such acceptability as "face validity."

Students find the OSCE to be a fairer alternative to traditional clinical examinations, as decisions in the OSCE are less prone to the subjective bias of the examiners. Examiners will accept the OSCE if the OSCE tests students on a wider range of physician competencies. Examiners may also find it reassuring that the pass/fail decision is not made by one individual; rather, it is made of the collective opinion of many learned examiners. The public and patients accept the OSCE as a better method for ensuring patient safety as the students have been tested on a range of practical and relevant competencies by a body of examiners.

Top three tips for improving the acceptability of the OSCE:

- Familiarize the students and faculty using a pilot OSCE run before the actual implementation.
- Collect focused feedback from students and faculty on the quality and appropriateness of the stations, with a view to meeting their expectations in the subsequent OSCEs.
- Choose only the practical and relevant competencies that students learned during their training, using an assessment blueprint.

Cost

The OSCE, like many other clinical examinations, is logistically challenging and can be a costly undertaking (Reznick *et al.*, 1993; Smee, 2003). The major costs of conducting an OSCE include the training of standardized patients, the payment of standardized patients during the examination, the costs associated with the arrangement of a venue, and the remuneration for examiners and examination administrators.

It may not be feasible for a single department or module (in a body system-based curriculum) to conduct an OSCE with a sufficient number of stations efficiently on a regular basis. We are of the view that departments or modules should combine their resources and conduct the OSCE jointly. Apart from sharing resources, this also creates an opportunity to develop an integrated examination.

Top three tips for improving the practicality and minimizing the resource utilization of the OSCE:

- Test only those competencies that cannot be tested by any other methods;
- Relegate components of competencies, such as spot diagnosis and interpretation of laboratory and radiological findings, to written assessments;
- Conduct combined OSCEs with other departments, modules, and even other institutions.

Summary

The OSCE's utility as an examination method can be addressed through proper consideration of its validity, reliability, educational impact, acceptability, and cost. Validity and reliability are psychometric considerations and other three factors are non-psychometric considerations. Validity is the most important consideration of a test. Adequate sampling is an essential element for improving the content validity and reliability of the OSCE. Educational impact, which can be either positive or negative, should always receive appropriate consideration during the test.

Answers to the self-learning exercise:

Factors	Possible Effects
Poorly trained standardized patients	Higher chance of variability in portraying patient findings
Poorly designed marking template	Misinterpretation of the marking criteria by the examiners
Inadequate station duration	Less opportunity to observe the candidate carefully
Vague instructions to examiners	Inconsistencies in marking
Vague instructions to candidates	Variable interpretation of the task within the station, leading to incomparable results
Vague instructions to patients	Patients acting differently with different candidates, leading to different candidates receiving a different (i.e. not the same) examination

References

Amin Z, Chong YS, Khoo HE. (2006) *Practical Guide to Medical Student Assessment*, 1st ed. World Scientific Publishing, Singapore.

Barman A. (2005) Critiques on the objective structured clinical examination. *Ann Acad Med Singapore* **34**(8): 478–482.

Downing SM. (2003) Validity: On the meaningful interpretation of assessment data. *Med Educ* **37**(9): 830–837.

Newble DI, Swansons DB. (1988) Psychometric characteristics of the objective structured clinical examination. *Med Educ* **22**(4): 325–334.

Newble DI. (1992) Assessing clinical competence at the undergraduate level. *Med Educ* **26**(6): 504–511.

Reznick RK, Smee SM, Buamber JS, Cohen R, Rothman AI, Blackmore DE, Berard M. (1993) Guidelines for estimating real cost of an objective structured clinical examination. *Acad Med* **68**(7): 513–517.

Smee S. (2003) ABC of teaching and learning in medicine: Skills based assessment. *Br Med J* **326**(7391): 703–706.

van der Vlueten CPM. (1996) The assessment of professional competence: Developments, research and practical implications. *Adv Health Sci Educ Theory Pract* **1**(1): 41–67.

4

SELECTING THE SKILLS TO BE TESTED IN AN OSCE THROUGH BLUEPRINTING

In Chapter 3, we discussed the importance of testing adequate and representative clinical competencies and content areas in the OSCE. Although the curriculum or the course itself details the clinical skills to be taught and learned, it is impossible to test all of the potential clinical skills to be assessed. How do we select clinical skills that can be tested? Is there a systematic way to sample an adequate number of clinical skills? The answers to these questions are fundamental to designing a good OSCE, and the most practical way of selecting a representative sample of skills to be tested is by developing an assessment blueprint.

At the end of this chapter, we should be able to:

(i) Recognize the importance of assessment blueprinting for enhancing the content validity of the OSCE.
(ii) Draw parallels between systematic sampling of research and systematic sampling in examination.
(iii) Analyze how an assessment blueprint can help us to plan an assessment system in order to evaluate a candidate's ability in a holistic manner.
(iv) Develop a master blueprint for an entire assessment.
(v) Develop a blueprint for an OSCE.

Basic Concepts of Blueprinting

An assessment process has to estimate how well a candidate has mastered "all" that has been taught and learnt. The latter (i.e. what has been taught and learnt) should be specified in the curriculum (McLaughlin, 2005; Coderre, Woloschuk & McLaughlin, 2009). A corollary to this assumption is that an ideal assessment system must assess the entire curriculum. However, this is not practical, primarily due to resource and logistical (e.g. time, examiners) constraints. Therefore, realistically speaking, any assessment can assess only a sample of a curriculum (Hamdy, 2006). An examination blueprint is a methodical process of sampling the learning outcomes (or competencies) and content of the curriculum. A blueprint defines what is to be tested in the examination and the weightage given to a specific area (Adkoli & Deepak, 2012) and suggests the best possible methods or tools of assessment.

Let us draw a corollary between sampling in research and sampling in examination. One of the cardinal rules in research dictates that the intended sample should be representative of the population from which the sample is obtained. Sampling in assessment is no different. In cases of assessment, the population represents the "curriculum" and the sample represents the "assessment". So, one of the most important rules in assessment is that assessment should represent the curriculum that it purports to test. This ensures the content validity (i.e. representativeness of the content) of the assessment.

Whether an assessment represents the curriculum that it purports to assess is determined by two criteria: adequacy and coverage of the assessment materials. Adequacy means that the amount of examination material included in the assessment should be sufficiently large. Not only should the examination material be adequate in size, but it should also cover most of the curriculum that it represents. This ensures that the candidate cannot pass the assessment without learning "all" as well as the "most" important parts of the curriculum. However, there is a tension between adequacy

👆 **Good to Know**

Adequacy versus coverage: Adequacy emphasizes that there should be a sufficiently large amount of examination materials included in the examination. However, these materials should not come from one or few areas. These examination materials should represent the entire curriculum, especially the important and critical elements that are needed to be a future doctor.

and coverage; i.e., the more the examiners attempt to cover the entire curriculum, the less likely that they can include material from any one area of the curriculum. How can these two opposing, but essential concepts of adequacy and coverage be reconciled? Blueprinting provides the answer.

In addition to addressing the adequacy and coverage of assessment materials, an assessment blueprint should also ensure that both the content and learning outcomes in the examination are proportionately represented with regards to the curriculum. This could be termed "proportionate coverage." Therefore, a blueprint, typically and in its most basic form, is a two-dimensional grid or table that meshes the curriculum content with the learning outcomes or competencies. Within this table (i.e. the blueprint), by convention, the rows represent the content, while the columns represent the learning outcomes (Newble, 2004). The assessment committee should ensure that each row and column is assessed either in the OSCE or in other examination formats. The number of times that a given content (row) or outcome (column) is assessed is determined by the principles of adequacy and coverage, as described earlier. In other words, blueprinting essentially follows a stratified sampling process, where the curriculum is stratified into its teaching and learning content (rows) and learning outcomes (columns).

Advantages of blueprints in an examination:

- A blueprint is an efficient method of test construction through scientific sampling (Hamdy, 2006);
- A blueprint reduces biases and guesswork;
- A blueprint drives faculty and students to focus on important aspects of the curriculum;
- A blueprint ensures that neglected, yet important, elements of the curriculum are adequately addressed;
- A blueprint brings greater transparency to the examination process (McLaughlin, 2005).

Master Blueprint

It is essential that we consider assessment not as a product of individual tools of assessment (such as MCQs, OSCEs, or workplace-based assessment) working in isolation, but as an assessment system comprising many such assessment tools working in synergy; i.e. complementing each other (Fig. 4.1). To this end, a master blueprint, which is for the entire assessment system, should be created before blueprinting each examination.

The steps of creating a master blueprint are as follows:

 (i) Draw a table;
 (ii) Include the learning outcomes of the curriculum that is to be assessed as columns;
(iii) Include the curriculum content as rows;
(iv) Identify how each cell that represents a given column and row can be assessed by assigning the appropriate assessment tool(s);
 (v) Complete Step (iv) for all of the cells.

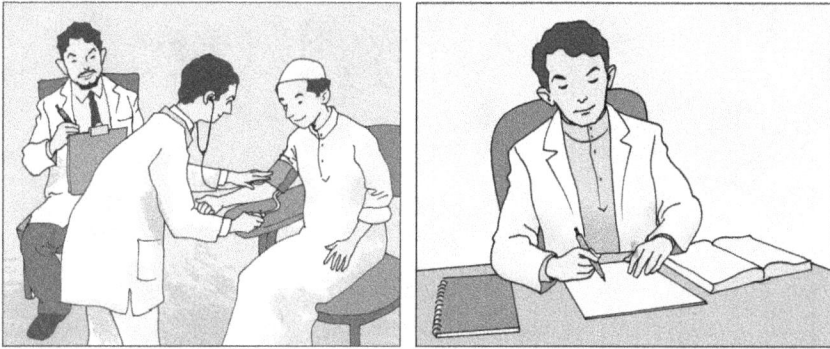

Fig. 4.1. The OSCE complements written assessment and generates a more holistic profile of a candidate.

Table 4.1 illustrates a master blueprint for a body system-based undergraduate curriculum. For simplicity, it is assumed that the assessment system only has three assessment tools: MCQ, OSCE, and a research project. Critically review how the cells in this blueprint have been filled. Please consider this only as an illustration, as there may be many other rational ways as to how the same cells could be filled.

Please note the following in the above master blueprint:

(i) All of the cells (or at least most of the cells) should be filled in with appropriate assessment tool(s);

(ii) One cell could accommodate more than one assessment tool;

(iii) The assessment tools should match the content and the learning outcome. For example, communication skills should not be assessed using MCQs. Hence, the column that represents communication skills does not have any cell that has MCQs as the assessment tool.

Table 4.1. A Master Blueprint Based on Saudi-Med Outcomes

Main learning Outcomes / Second-level outcomes (competencies)	Scientific Approach		Patient Care					Community Orientation		Communication and Collaboration			Professionalism			Research
	Integration of basic sciences	Evidence-based medicine	Clinical skills	Clinical reasoning	Management of critical conditions	Management of common conditions	Patient-centered care	Healthcare system	Health promotion and disease prevention	Teamwork	Communication skills	Information technology	Attitudes and behavior	Moral and ethical principles	Professional development and self-regulation	Basic research skills
Cardiovascular system	MCQ	MCQ	OSCE	OSCE	OSCE / MCQ	MCQ / OSCE	MCQ / OSCE	MCQ	MCQ / OSCE	OSCE	OSCE	Project	OSCE	OSCE / MCQ	Project / MCQ	Project / MCQ
Respiratory system	MCQ	OSCE	OSCE	MCQ	MCQ	MCQ / OSCE	MCQ / OSCE	MCQ / OSCE	MCQ / OSCE	OSCE	OSCE	Project	OSCE	OSCE / MCQ	OSCE / Project	Project / MCQ
Gastrointestinal system	MCQ	MCQ	OSCE	OSCE	MCQ	MCQ	MCQ	MCQ	MCQ	OSCE	OSCE	Project	OSCE	OSCE	Project	Project
Immune system	MCQ	MCQ	OSCE	MCQ	MCQ	MCQ	MCQ	MCQ	MCQ	OSCE	OSCE	Project	OSCE	OSCE	Project	Project
Locomotor system	MCQ	MCQ	OSCE	OSCE	MCQ	MCQ / OSCE	MCQ / OSCE	MCQ	MCQ / OSCE	OSCE	OSCE	Project	OSCE	OSCE / MCQ	Project / MCQ	Project / MCQ
Endocrine system	MCQ	MCQ	OSCE	MCQ	MCQ	MCQ / OSCE	MCQ / OSCE	MCQ	MCQ / OSCE	OSCE	OSCE	Project	OSCE	OSCE / MCQ	Project / MCQ	Project / MCQ
Nervous system	MCQ	MCQ	OSCE	OSCE	MCQ	MCQ	MCQ	MCQ	MCQ	OSCE	OSCE	Project	OSCE	OSCE	Project	Project

(Continued)

Table 4.1. (*Continued*)

Main learning Outcomes / Second-level outcomes (competencies)	Scientific Approach			Patient Care				Community Orientation		Communication and Collaboration			Professionalism			Research
	Integration of basic sciences	Evidence-based medicine	Clinical skills	Clinical reasoning	Management of critical conditions	Management of common conditions	Patient-centered care	Healthcare system	Health promotion and disease prevention	Teamwork	Communication skills	Information technology	Attitudes and behavior	Moral and ethical principles	Professional development and self-regulation	Basic research skills
Reproductive system	MCQ	MCQ	OSCE	MCQ	MCQ	MCQ	MCQ	MCQ	MCQ	OSCE	OSCE	Project	OSCE	OSCE	Project	Project
Genitourinary system	MCQ	MCQ	OSCE	OSCE	MCQ	MCQ	MCQ	MCQ	MCQ	OSCE	OSCE	Project	OSCE	OSCE	Project	Project
Growth and development	MCQ OSCE	MCQ	OSCE	MCQ OSCE	MCQ	MCQ OSCE	MCQ OSCE	MCQ	MCQ OSCE	OSCE	OSCE	Project	OSCE	OSCE MCQ	Project MCQ	Project MCQ
Elderly care	MCQ	OSCE	OSCE	OSCE	MCQ	MCQ	MCQ	MCQ	MCQ	OSCE	OSCE	Project	OSCE	OSCE	Project	Project
Infectious diseases	MCQ	MCQ	OSCE	MCQ	MCQ	MCQ	MCQ	MCQ	MCQ	OSCE	OSCE	Project	OSCE	OSCE	Project	Project
Multi-system diseases	MCQ	MCQ	OSCE	MCQ	MCQ OSCE	MCQ OSCE	MCQ OSCE	MCQ OSCE	MCQ OSCE	OSCE	OSCE	Project	OSCE	OSCE MCQ	Project MCQ	Project MCQ

OSCE Blueprint

It is only once the master blueprint is created that the sampling process begins. So, if the OSCE blueprint is to be formulated using the above master blueprint, then the OSCE components of this master blueprint need to be extracted. Thereafter, out of the cells that are tagged as OSCE, consider sampling an appropriate number of cells that would ensure adequacy and coverage.

Table 4.2 illustrates such an OSCE blueprint. Ticks in this blueprint denote the selected (or the sampled) assessment content for a given administration of the OSCE.

In this blueprint, the following should be emphasized:

(i) Each tick could represent either one OSCE station or several OSCE stations in order to ensure the adequacy of the assessment of the curriculum;

(ii) Similarly, several ticks can represent one OSCE station in order to ensure coverage of the curriculum. This is a particularly important concept for the development of integrated stations;

(iii) All columns and rows that have been tagged as OSCE have been ticked (i.e. selected) at least once.

Hence, depending on the relative importance of the assessment content and outcome, one or many stations can be included in the OSCE to represent a given cell, while at the same time ensuring the coverage of the curriculum.

The next step is to convert the preliminary blueprint shown in Table 4.2 to a proper OSCE blueprint. For this step, the cells (i.e. the content and learning outcomes) selected through the sampling process illustrated in Table 4.2 should be transformed into OSCE stations. One example of such a conversion using the sampling process initiated in Table 4.2 into OSCE stations is shown in Table 4.3. Note that in Table 4.3, one tick in Table 4.2 may sometimes imply one station or more than one station; e.g. Station 1 and Station 2 (S1 and S2) in the cell with the coordinates of cardiovascular system and patient-centered care. Similarly, sometimes several ticks in Table 4.2 represent only one station in Table 4.3; e.g. S3.

Table 4.2. Preliminary OSCE Blueprint

Main learning Outcomes	Scientific Approach		Patient Care					Community Orientation		Communication and Collaboration			Professionalism			Research
Second-level outcomes (competencies)	Integration of basic sciences	Evidence-based medicine	Clinical skills	Clinical reasoning	Management of critical conditions	Management of common conditions	Patient-centered care	Healthcare system	Health promotion and disease prevention	Teamwork	Communication skills	Information technology	Attitudes and behavior	Moral and ethical principles	Professional development and self-regulation	Basic research skills
Cardiovascular system			OSCE	OSCE	OSCE	OSCE	OSCE		OSCE	OSCE	OSCE		OSCE	OSCE		
Respiratory system		OSCE	OSCE		OSCE	OSCE	OSCE	OSCE	OSCE	OSCE	OSCE		OSCE	OSCE	OSCE	
Gastrointestinal system			OSCE	OSCE						OSCE	OSCE		OSCE	OSCE		
Immune system			OSCE			OSCE	OSCE			OSCE	OSCE		OSCE	OSCE		
Locomotor system			OSCE	OSCE		OSCE	OSCE		OSCE	OSCE	OSCE		OSCE	OSCE		
Endocrine system			OSCE			OSCE	OSCE		OSCE	OSCE	OSCE		OSCE	OSCE		
Nervous system			OSCE	OSCE					OSCE	OSCE	OSCE		OSCE	OSCE		
Reproductive system			OSCE							OSCE	OSCE		OSCE	OSCE		

(*Continued*)

Table 4.2.   (*Continued*)

Main learning Outcomes	Scientific Approach		Patient Care					Community Orientation		Communication and Collaboration			Professionalism			Research
Second-level outcomes (competencies)	Integration of basic sciences	Evidence-based medicine	Clinical skills	Clinical reasoning	Management of critical conditions	Management of common conditions	Patient-centered care	Healthcare system	Health promotion and disease prevention	Teamwork	Communication skills	Information technology	Attitudes and behavior	Moral and ethical principles	Professional development and self-regulation	Basic research skills
Genitourinary system	OSCE✓		OSCE✓	OSCE						OSCE	OSCE		OSCE✓	OSCE		
Growth and development	OSCE✓		OSCE	OSCE		OSCE	OSCE✓		OSCE	OSCE	OSCE		OSCE	OSCE		
Elderly care		OSCE✓	OSCE	OSCE✓						OSCE	OSCE		OSCE✓	OSCE		
Infectious diseases			OSCE							OSCE	OSCE✓		OSCE	OSCE		
Multi-system diseases	OSCE✓		OSCE✓			OSCE	OSCE	OSCE✓	OSCE✓	OSCE✓	OSCE		OSCE	OSCE	OSCE	

Table 4.3. Final OSCE Blueprint

Main learning Outcomes	Scientific Approach		Patient Care					Community Orientation		Communication and Collaboration			Professionalism			Research
Second-level outcomes (competencies)	Integration of basic sciences	Evidence-based medicine	Clinical skills	Clinical reasoning	Management of critical conditions	Management of common conditions	Patient-centered care	Healthcare system	Health promotion and disease prevention	Teamwork	Communication skills	Information technology	Attitudes and behavior	Moral and ethical principles	Professional development and self-regulation	Basic research skills
Cardiovascular system			S1		S2		S1,2									
Respiratory system						S3			S3						S3	
Gastrointestinal system			S4										S4			
Immune system										S5						
Locomotor system						S6								S6		
Endocrine system			S7								S7		S7			
Nervous system				S8							S9					

(Continued)

Table 4.3. (*Continued*)

Main learning Outcomes	Scientific Approach		Patient Care					Community Orientation		Communication and Collaboration			Professionalism			Research
Second-level outcomes (competencies)	Integration of basic sciences	Evidence-based medicine	Clinical skills	Clinical reasoning	Management of critical conditions	Management of common conditions	Patient-centered care	Healthcare system	Health promotion and disease prevention	Teamwork	Communication skills	Information technology	Attitudes and behavior	Moral and ethical principles	Professional development and self-regulation	Basic research skills
Reproductive system											S10					
Genitourinary system			S11										S11			
Growth and development							S12									
Elderly care		S13		S13										S13		
Infectious diseases									S15		S14					
Multi-system diseases	S12		S15					S15	S15	S15						

Alternatively, although not ideal, you might want to develop a simplified blueprint for an OSCE. Here, we shall critically review two other simpler blueprints; the first one (Table 4.4) is for the final exit (Final MBBS) examination of an undergraduate program, and the second (Table 4.5) is for a specific course. Typically, you should start by specifying the tasks of the physicians on the top row and domains or body system on the left-most column. Then, you start choosing the clinical tasks that you would like to include in the grid.

Let us review the blueprint for the exit examination (Table 4.4) first. The top-most row details the typical tasks to be carried out in the OSCE. The left-most column details the major body systems. The second column specifies the presenting problem. The third column specifies the context of practice, whereas the fourth column specifies gender and age group. These specifications are important for minimizing the bias towards in-patients and adult male patients, which is typical of clinical examinations. You might choose to have other specifications. The numbers (1, 2, 3, etc) represent the OSCE station. Numbers in bold indicate the primary emphasis of the OSCE station. For example, in the smoking cessation station (Station 1), the primary emphasis will be health promotion and health prevention, while communication and counselling and professionalism are of ancillary importance.

A second example of an OSCE blueprint is for the end-of-course or rotation examination. Many medical schools conduct such OSCEs after the end of their clinical rotations. This particular example (Table 4.5) is developed for an end-of-rotation of the psychiatry posting. This is a very simplified version that is based on competency and major groups of disorders in psychiatry.

Table 4.4. A Simplified Blueprint for the Exit Examination (Final MBBS) in an Undergraduate Program (please note, other body systems should also be included in the blueprint)

Body System	Presenting Problem	Context of Practice	Gender and Age Group	Health Promotion and Prevention	History Taking	Physical Examination	Investigation	Diagnosis	Management	Communication and Counselling	Professionalism
Healthy individual	Smoking Cessation	Community	Adult male	1						1	1
	Life-style modification	Out-patient	Adult male	2	2					2	
Abdomen	Acute abdomen	Emergency	Adult female		3	3		3			
	Jaundice	In-patient	Child				4		4		
	Upper gastrointestinal bleed	Emergency	Adult male		5			5	5		4
Respiratory	Prolonged cough	Out-patient	Adult female		6	6	6				
	Common cold	Out-patient	Adult female		7	7					7

Table 4.5. A Simplified Blueprint for an End-of-rotation OSCE in Psychiatry (please note, other major groups of disorders should also be included in the blueprint)

Psychiatric Disorder	Gender and Age group	History Taking and Physical Examination	Diagnosis	Medication	Management	Patient and Family Education	Communication and Counselling	Professionalism
Anxiety disorders	Female, middle age	1	1	1				
Depressions	Male, middle age		2		2		2	
Eating disorders	Female, adolescent	3				3	3	
Personality disorders	Male, middle age		4		4			4
Psychosis	Male, middle age			5		5	5	
Substance abuse	Male, middle age			6		6		6
Suicide	Female, old age	7			7		7	

Further Specifications

Apart from curricular content and learning outcomes, it might be worthwhile to have further specifications, as depicted in Tables 4.4 and 4.5, in the assessment in general and the OSCE in particular. Further specifications may include the relative distribution of stations between sites of care, gender, age, nature of clinical problems, and priority of the problems in the community.

Site of Care

Although the vast majority of encounters between healthcare providers and patients take place out of the hospital, typical clinical examinations are heavily skewed towards in-patient medical problems. Research from Green *et al.* (2001) provides us with robust evidence of the importance of considering the site of care in the sampling of stations. Simply speaking, if we follow 1000 persons in the community for a month, about 800 persons would report some kind of symptoms. Of these, 327 persons would seek some form of medical care; most of this medical care would take place in the out-of-hospital setting. Out of the initial 1000 persons, only eight persons would be hospitalized and less than one (<0.1%) of them would be hospitalized in an academic healthcare center. It is ironic that the majority of the clinical materials tested in the examination are from the minority hospitalized patients.

Therefore, it is imperative that the examination planner provides some guidance to the test developers regarding the relative distribution of stations from the various sites of care, such as in-patient, out-patient, acute care, and the community, among others. Table 4.6 shows a suggested distribution with examples of representative tasks to be performed.

Age and Gender of the Patients

The OSCE should ensure that the age and gender of the patients represented in the examination reflect the larger society. There should not be an over- or under-representation of a specific age group. Below is an example of age distributions (Table 4.7).

Nature of Clinical Problems

It is imperative that the OSCE blueprint should be reviewed in order to ensure that the stations represent important clinical conditions. While the majority of the stations should come from common conditions, a small proportion may also come from uncommon and illustrative conditions. It might be useful to

Table 4.6. Suggested Distribution of OSCE Stations According to Site of Care

Site of Care	Proportion of OSCE Stations	Example of Tasks in the OSCE
In-patient	~20–30%	"You are the doctor assessing a patient who has been recently hospitalized for respiratory distress. Examine his respiratory system."
Out-patient	~30–40%	"Mrs. Hamid, a 30-year-old previously healthy patient, comes to the clinic with a headache. Take a history from Mrs. Hamid."
Acute care	~10–20%	"A 21-year-old man was brought in to the emergency room following a road-traffic accident. Take a handover from the emergency medical technician."
Community	~10–20%	"You are the medical officer posted to a village. Deliver a brief talk to the school children on the dangers of cigarette smoking."

Table 4.7. Suggested Distribution of OSCE Stations According to Age and Gender

Age Group	Relative Distribution of Stations in the OSCE
Newborn and pediatric	~10–20%
Adolescent and youth	~10–20%
Adult	~50–60%
Elderly	~20–30%

prioritize the clinical presentation of the OSCE stations into one of the following four categories:

- Common;
- Curable;
- Preventable;
- Life-, limb-, vision-saving.

Summary

It is our collective observation that the blueprint is often neglected in examination planning. In our view, the blueprint is the only feasible and practical method for ensuring proper sampling of the examination. The blueprint improves the content validity of the examination, provides transparency to candidates and examiners regarding the examination, ensures fair representation of content and learning outcomes, and makes the process of station development rigorous. The master blueprint ensures holistic sampling of candidates' competencies and content areas with appropriate assessment instruments. The OSCE-specific blueprint is derived from the master blueprint and is customized to the examination. Once the OSCE blueprint is drawn, it is important that the fulfillment of the further specifications, such as the site of care, age, gender, and nature of problems, is checked within the OSCE blueprint in order to ensure the realistic portrayal of patients' problems within different settings and demographic parameters.

References

Adkoli BV, Deepak KK. (2012) Blueprinting in assessment. In: Singh T, Anshu (eds), *Principles of Assessment in Medical Education*, Jaypee Brothers Medical Publishers, India, pp. 205–213.

Coderre S, Woloschuk W, McLaughlin K. (2009) Twelve tips for blueprinting. *Med Teach* **31**(4): 22–324.

Green LA, Yawn BP, Lanier D, Dovey SM. (2001) The ecology of medical care revisited. *N Engl J Med* **344**(26): 2021–2025.

Hamdy H. (2006) Blueprinting for assessment of healthcare professionals. *Clin Teach* **3**: 175–179.

McLaughlin K, Coderre S, Woloschuk W, Mandin H. (2005) Does blueprint publication affect students' perception of validity of the evaluation process? *Adv Health Sci Educ Theory Pract* **10**(1): 15–22.

McLaughlin K, Lemaire J, Coderre S. (2005) Creating a reliable and valid blueprint for the internal medicine clerkship evaluation. *Med Teach* **27**(6): 544–547.

Newble D. (2004) Techniques for measuring clinical competence: Objective structured clinical examinations. *Med Educ* **38**(2): 199–203.

5

UTILIZING DIFFERENT FORMATS OF OSCE FOR GREATER EFFICIENCY

As mentioned in previous chapters, the OSCE is a multi-task, multi-station, multi-examiner assessment method that assesses skills of history taking, clinical examination, communication, and procedural skills (Boursicot & Roberts, 2005). However, within its basic tenants, the OSCE continues to serve different purposes with varied formats. The OSCE formats may differ according to the purpose of assessment, the course objectives, and among different specialties. As an examiner and OSCE planner, you should be able to utilize different OSCE formats to suit your needs.

At the end of this chapter, we should be able to:

(i) Review different formats of OSCE.
(ii) Determine how the purpose and context of a given situation determine the format of an OSCE.
(iii) Examine the relative merits of different OSCE formats.
(iv) Select the OSCE formats to suit the needs of a given situation.

Formative and Summative OSCEs

A formative OSCE, as the name suggests, is primarily for supporting student learning. In addition, a formative OSCE might be used for the orientation of students and staff, especially when an OSCE is to be introduced for the first time as a summative assessment.

The OSCE can also be used as a structured teaching tool (Adamo, 2003). Formative OSCEs also have the potential to improve students' competence during a summative OSCE (Townsend *et al.*, 2001).

OSCEs can support learning by various means, including structured feedback during or after the OSCE, review of examiners' comments regarding the candidates, and review of the captured videos of the candidates. If feedback is to be included in the OSCE, it is essential that systematic data collection about the candidates' competence is included in the marking scheme in the form of itemized marking and/or qualitative comments.

The summative OSCE is the main OSCE format. A summative OSCE is conducted at the end of a course, a clinical attachment, or for the purposes of final certification. A summative OSCE is a high-stakes examination where major decisions are made regarding a candidate's ability to function as a doctor. Notwithstanding its main purpose, it is recommended that elements of feedback are included at the end of a summative OSCE, either in the form of a group debriefing or one-to-one feedback.

Active and Static Stations

The OSCE stations can be also classified into active and static stations. Active stations contain patient/SP encounters in order to assess the skills of focused interview/history taking, clinical examination, communication, and/or procedural skills (Fig. 5.1). Static stations are used also to assess the candidate's ability to interpret laboratory data, radiological images, clinical photographs, and other relevant materials such as electrocardiograms (ECGs), electroencephalograms (EEGs), and growth charts. No examiner or SP/patient is required in such types of station (Fig. 5.2). Our recommendation is to test the latter abilities through written or computer-based testing, especially when they are not linked to another manned station. This would reduce the time and resources needed and hence more active stations could be included in the OSCE (Fig. 5.2).

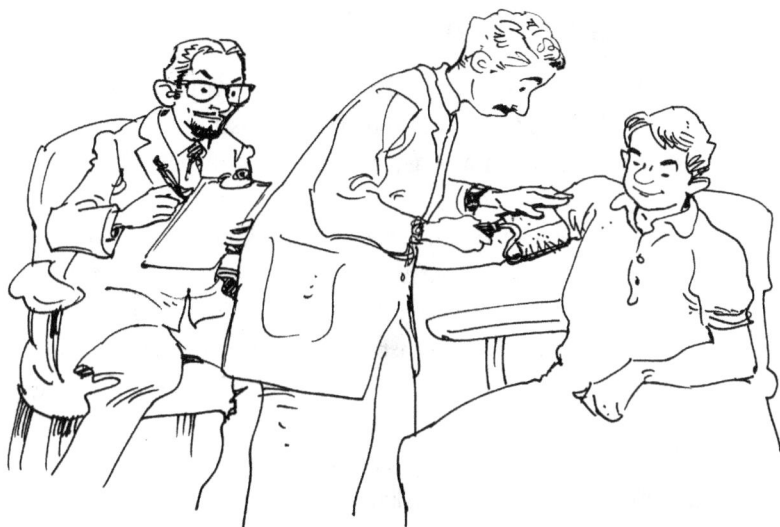

Fig. 5.1. An OSCE station should include clinical tasks.

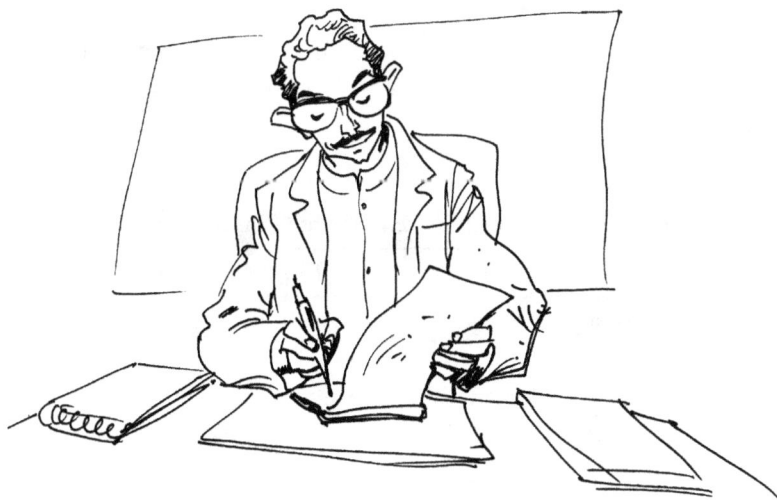

Fig. 5.2. Many elements of static stations can be tested through written examinations.

Couplet or Linked Stations

In some situations, not all of the desired competencies can be assessed in one OSCE station due to time constraints or the nature of the tasks. In such situations, additional competencies can be assessed in an adjacent station — a feature known as couplet or linked stations. The use of linked stations extends the number of tasks that can be completed within a given activity. For example, an OSCE station could be developed in order to assess a candidate's competence in performing breast examination. A second station could assess the candidate's ability to communicate the findings to the patient.

Linked stations (Table 5.1) are attractive as they tend to preserve the wholeness of the tasks. However, a large number of linked stations reduces the content coverage. Furthermore, students may be penalized in the second station for mistakes committed while at the first station. It is our recommendation to reserve linked stations for specialized tasks and not to use too many linked stations in a given OSCE.

The OSCE circuit needs to be configured differently if linked stations are to be included. The configuration of linked stations is shown in Fig. 5.3.

Table 5.1.　Possible Scenarios for Linked Stations

First Station	Linked Second Station
Take a history of a patient with breathlessness	Perform a focused cardiorespiratory examination
Do a pre-operative assessment of a surgical patient	Explain the intended surgical procedure to the patient
Assess a patient with newly diagnosed diabetes	Teach the patient and caregiver the proper use of medications
Assess the gait of an elderly patient with stroke	Counsel the family regarding fall-prevention strategies

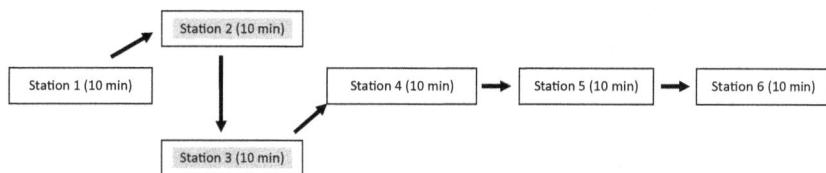

Fig. 5.3. Incorporating linked stations within a standard OSCE with 10-minute stations.

At the beginning of the OSCE circuit, Station 3 should be vacant; i.e. without a candidate. Alternatively, the first candidate in Station 2 should start the OSCE 10 minutes before the other candidates. This is because Station 3 cannot be attempted by a candidate without completing Station 2.

Long-Station OSCEs

The purpose of a long-station (double station) is to assess clinical skills comprehensively in each station. The duration of a station is much longer than a traditional OSCE station. The long-station OSCE is configured to assess history taking, physical examination, data interpretation, diagnosis, communication, and management with real or simulated patients (Dacre *et al.*, 2006).

The major pitfall of long-station OSCEs is that each station takes 30–60 min to complete, thereby restricting the domains or clinical skills to be tested in an examination. If a long-station OSCE is to be used, it must be supplemented by adequate numbers of other OSCE stations in order to capture a range of competencies.

How can we incorporate long stations within a standard OSCE circuit? Suppose, in a given OSCE, the duration of each standard station is 10 min. However, there is one task (e.g., comprehensive psychiatric assessment) that would require 20 minutes to complete. Moreover, the task cannot be broken down into two subtasks, and thereby tested through two linked stations. The following design strategies (Figs. 5.3 and 5.4) would allow us to incorporate a longer OSCE station within the standard OSCE circuit in the form of a double or triple station.

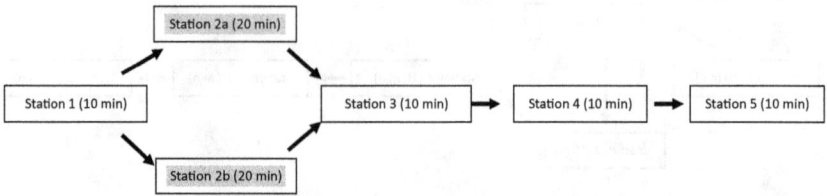

Fig. 5.4. Incorporating a 20-minute station within a standard OSCE with 10-minute stations.

Note that Stations 2a and 2b will not start at the same time. At the beginning of the circuit, a candidate (candidate A) will be assigned to Station 2a and Station 2b will remain without any candidate. Ten minutes later, the candidate in Station 1 (candidate B), after completing Station 1, will proceed to Station 2b. The candidate in Station 2a (candidate A) will continue with the assigned task. After another 10 minutes (i.e. 20 minutes after the start of the circuit), the candidate in Station 2a (candidate A) completes their task and is ready to move to Station 3, whereas the candidate in Station 2b (candidate B) still continues with their task. Another candidate (candidate C), now in Station 1, will replace the first candidate in Station 2a (candidate A), who will leave for Station 3.

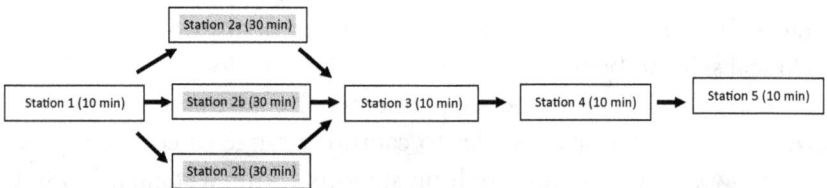

Fig. 5.5. Incorporating a 30-minute station within a standard OSCE with 10-minute stations.

Objective Structured Practical Examination

The Objective Structured Practical Examination (OSPE) is also a multi-station examination format that is particularly suited for basic medical science assessment (Dissanayake, Ali & Nayar, 1990).

However, instead of testing clinical skills, the focus of the OSPE is primarily on practical and interpretative skills that cannot be tested in written tests. The OSPE is suitable for integrated curricula and cheaper than traditional practical examinations (Feroze & Jacob, 2002; Yaqinuddin *et al.*, 2013).

In the OSPE, the station duration tends to be shorter and many more stations are included in the circuit. As the OSPE is conducted in a large open room, typically only two to three examiners are needed for the entire session. This is possible because most OSPE stations are not manned (i.e. not active) stations. The OSPE examiners do not need intensive briefing like in the OSCE; however, they should be familiar with the examination format and materials (Zafar *et al.*, 2013). Table 5.2 shows the differences between the OSPE and the OSCE.

Table 5.2.   Differences Between the OSPE and the OSCE in Assessment (Feroze & Jacob, 2002; Yaqinuddin *et al.*, 2013)

OSPE in Basic Sciences	OSCE in Basic Sciences
Primary objective is to test the identification and interpretation of data	Primary objective is to test the application of basic sciences knowledge to a patient or a normal person
Examples of materials used: Cadaver, prosected or dissected specimens, gross pathology, histopathology, radiological images, pharmacokinetic properties of drugs, etc	Examples of tasks: Application of the ECG leads on the precordium, palpation of the external inguinal orifice, estimation of peak expiration flow rate, measuring blood pressure, etc
Tests clinical relevance	Tests clinical application
No direct observation is needed by an examiner	Examiners are needed
Less time is needed per station; typical station duration is 3–5 minutes	More time is needed per station; typical station duration is 8–10 minutes

Conventional OSCEs can also be employed to test relevant clinical skills and the application of basic sciences knowledge in early undergraduate years. This might be particularly attractive for a vertically integrated curriculum where clinical relevance and application feature prominently in the first 2–3 years of medical school. Table 5.3 lists some of the examples of skills that are relevant to early medical school years and that can be tested in the OSCE and that are relevant to early undergraduate years.

Table 5.3. Examples of Skills that are Relevant to the Early Years of Medical School that can be Tested in the OSCE

Basic Sciences Knowledge	Corresponding Clinical Applications that can be Tested in the OSCE
Surface anatomy of abdominal viscera	Abdominal examination
Function of cranial nerves	Cranial nerve examination
Relationship between prostate and surrounding structures	Digital per-rectal examination
Biological function of glucose-6-phosphate dehydrogenase (G6PD)	Counsel families regarding the pathogenesis and clinical implications of G6PD deficiency
Carbohydrate metabolism	Explain pathogenesis of diabetes to a patient

Summary

The OSCE can be of many different formats depending on the purposes of the assessment and context of the given clinical scenario. The OSCE may be formative or summative in nature, although consideration for the improvement of learning should always be taken into account regardless of whether the OSCE is formative or summative. The OSCE should not be misused in order to test components of knowledge that can be assessed in a written test; rather, the OSCE should be reserved for assessing clinical competencies that cannot be tested by paper-and-pencil examinations or computer-based testing formats. The inclusion of non-standard OSCE formats, such as long-station OSCEs or linked stations, should be based on careful consideration of the needs for such stations and the impact of such an inclusion on the overall examination.

References

Adamo G. (2003) Simulated and standardized patients in OSCEs: Achievements and challenges 1992–2003. *Med Teach* **425(3)**: 262–270.

Boursicot K, Roberts T. (2005) How to set up an OSCE. *Clin Teach* 2(1):16–20.

Dacre J, Gaffan J, Dunkley L, Sturrock A. 2006. A new final clinical examination. *Clin Teach* 3(1): 29–33.

Dissanayake AS, Ali BA, Nayar U. (1990) The influence of the introduction of objective structured practical examinations in physiology on student performance at King Faisal University Medical School. *Med Teach* 12(3–4): 297–304.

Feroze M, Jacob AJ. (2002) OSPE in pathology. *Indian J Pathol Microbiol* 45: 53–58.

Townsend AH, McIlvenny S, Miller CJ, Dunn EV. (2001) The use of an Objective Structured Clinical Examination (OSCE) for formative and summative assessment in a general practice clinical attachment and its relationship to final medical school examination performance. *Med Educ* 35(9): 841–846.

Yaqinuddin A, Zafar M, Ikram MF, Ganguly P. (2013) What is an objective structured practical examination in anatomy? *Anat Sci Educ* 6(2): 125–133.

Zafar M, Yaqinuddin A, Ikram MF, Ganguly P. (2013) Practical examination: OSPE, OSCE and spots. In: Ganguly P (ed.), *Education in Anatomical Sciences*. Nova Biomedical, NY, pp. 223–237.

6

WRITING OSCE STATIONS

The OSCE blueprint, discussed in Chapter 4, provides us with a list of competencies and content areas to be tested in the examination. We have already discussed the importance of developing the master blueprint and the OSCE-specific blueprint. The next step is to write the OSCE station according to the description provided in the blueprint.

At the end of this chapter, we should be able to:

(i) Adopt a structured approach to developing OSCE stations.
(ii) Develop skills to implement the OSCE.
(iii) Systematically review prototypes of checklists and instructions in order to customize and develop the OSCE for the required purposes.

Forming the Team to Write the OSCE Station

Once the OSCE blueprint has been finalized, the OSCE Committee or the Examination Committee should delegate the responsibility of developing individual OSCE stations to an interdisciplinary team, typically representing the specialties that are to be tested. Let us review the final OSCE blueprint (Table 4.3; page 47). Station 3 is related to the respiratory system and has three learning outcomes: Management of common clinical conditions, health promotion and disease prevention, and professional development and self-regulation. The Station 3 team might consist of representatives from respiratory medicine, family medicine, and the ethics and professionalism track, with the respiratory medicine specialist taking the role of the leader. It is our strong recommendation that OSCE stations need to be developed in an interdisciplinary manner in order to promote integration and contextualization and to minimize the potential bias of any particular discipline.

The OSCE station writing team is responsible for developing the following:

(i) Instructions to the candidate;
(ii) Instructions to the standardized patient/simulated patient;
(iii) Instructions to the examiners;
(iv) Preparing a list of equipment or materials needed for the examination;
(v) Creating a scoring template.

In this chapter, our focus will be on the first four of these responsibilities. The scoring template, which deserves a more in-depth discussion, will be dealt with in the next chapter.

Developing Instructions to the Candidate

Instructions to the candidate should contain following information:

(i) A brief background of the patient or the condition;
(ii) The tasks to be performed by the candidate;
(iii) Any restrictions or limitations;
(iv) The station duration;
(v) Any other special instructions, such as:

(a) Who will be marking the candidate — examiners or standardized patients;
(b) Whether examiners will ask questions from the candidate;

(c) Whether the candidate is supposed to present the findings either in writing or verbally to the examiners;

(d) Whether this is a linked or double station.

Instructions to the candidate need to be precise, clear, and focused. Let us compare two examples of instructions to the candidate. This is meant to be a counseling and communication station. Ahmad is a 3-year-old boy with recently diagnosed asthma. The candidate's task is to counsel the parents regarding proper use of the metered dose inhaler using a face mask.

Example A

Station 5
Instructions to the candidate

Ahmad is a 3-year-old boy with asthma. Please talk to the mother and respond to her concerns.

Example B

Station 5
Instructions to the candidate

This is a counseling/communication station.

Ahmad is a 3-year-old boy with recently diagnosed asthma. Please enter the room and counsel Ahmad's mother regarding the use of the metered dose inhaler and facemask and respond to her questions. You are expected to interact only with Ahmad's mother.

You have 8 minutes to complete this task.

In Example A, there is a possibility that the candidate would misinterpret the instructions and may start taking a history related to Ahmad's asthma. Unless the standardized patient (Ahmad's mother) is particularly skillful, there is a chance that the station might not function as expected, with the candidate spending more time in taking a history of Ahmad's asthma rather than counseling the mother in the use of a metered dose inhaler, which was the original intention of the station.

In Example B, relevant background information is provided to the candidate with clearer instructions and the expected tasks to be performed by the candidate. Let us look at some of the key words in Example B and the reasons for their inclusion.

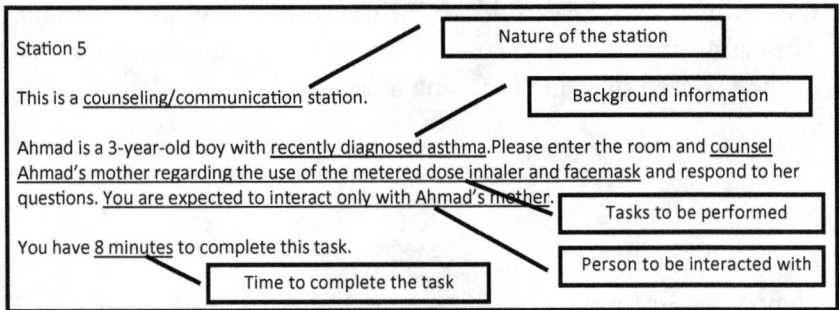

Developing Instructions to the Simulated and Standardized Patients

Simulated patients or standardized patients may include actors, lay persons, or real patients with stable medical conditions (Adamo, 2003; Cleland, Abe, & Rethan, 2009). In this chapter, we have used "SP" to denote both simulated and standardized patients.

Instructions to the simulated patient should be detailed (Amin, Chong & Khoo, 2006; van der Vleuten & Swanson 1990). It may need several rounds of training and pilot testing before finalizing the simulated patient for the main examination.

The information that may need to be included will depend on the nature of the station and the task(s) to be performed. Information might include:

- A brief description of the condition or case to be portrayed;
- Tasks to be performed by the candidate;
- The role of the simulated patients;
- The opening statement, if any, by the simulated patients;
- Expected questions from the candidate and suggested answers;

- The demeanor of the simulated patients;
- List of dos and don'ts.

Below is an abbreviated example of instructions to simulated patients. You might want to create a more detailed version depending on your needs. This is a psychiatry station in which the candidate's task is to take a history from a patient who suffers from generalized anxiety disorder. Today, the patient presents with a fear of riding on elevators. Note that, in this station, the SP is not required to assess the candidate.

Example of simulated patient instructions

Background information

- Name: Madam Sufia
- Age: 25 years
- Marital status: Single
- Education: University graduate
- Employment: Office administrator
- Language requirement: Bilingual, able to communicate in English
- Premorbid condition: None
- Current medication: None
- Associated medical/surgical condition: None
- Set-up: General practitioner's office

Competencies to be tested in this station
This station will assess candidate's ability to:

- Obtain a focused history of a patient with generalized anxiety disorder
- Use verbal and nonverbal communication effectively in a medical set-up

Purpose of the visit
You have come to the doctor's office to consult him/her about your fear

SP's role

- Your role is limited to portraying the patient scenario faithfully
- You are not required to assess the candidate
- You should not provide feedback on the candidate's performance to the examiner
- Do not volunteer any information unless asked by the candidate

(Continued)

(*Continued*)

Description of the problem
You have been suffering from intense fear whenever you come near an elevator. This has been going on for the last 3 years. However, the fear has been getting more intense during the last couple of months. You feel that this has affected your office work and social life. Your office is on the 15th floor. Several times a day you have to take the elevator to meet other office co-workers. Occasionally, you avoid riding on the elevator altogether.

Recently, you have been on a family vacation. You were given room on the 21st floor. You could not stay in that hotel because of your fear of taking the elevator. This has created a very embarrassing situation for you.

Characteristics of attacks

- Breathing difficulty
- Palpitations
- Choking sensation
- Trembling of hands
- Sweating, especially on palms and soles
- Feeling of throwing up

The attacks are not associated with hearing strange voices or seeing visions. Nobody tries to manipulate your thoughts or behaviors. You cannot remember any specific event that led to this anxiety. You do not remember any significant childhood mental trauma or abuse.

If asked, state the followings:
- No suicidal thoughts
- No depression
- No other family member has similar symptoms

Demeanor
You should appear anxious without being overtly depressed. You should be able to make good eye contact and communicate clearly.

Respond to the candidate with short phrases if the candidate asks closed-ended questions.

Respond to the candidate more elaborately if the candidate asks open-ended questions.

If unsure, your response should be "I don't feel like talking about it," or "I don't remember clearly."

Developing Instructions to the Examiners

Like the instructions for the students, instructions for the examiners need to be very carefully scrutinized and reviewed before the actual examination (Selby *et al.*, 1995). In addition, the examiners should have access to the instructions that are given to the candidate and to the SPs. It is imperative that examiners are instructed to follow the agreed-upon checklists and criteria while examining students, leaving aside their personal preferences and biases (Selby *et al.*, 1995).

Depending on the case, typical instructions to the examiners may include:

- The nature of the stations;
- The tasks to be performed by the candidate;
- The findings of the patient/mannequins;
- The expected level of competency required to pass the station;
- The difficulty level of the station;
- The role of examiners during the OSCE.

Recommended practice

- Make sure that the instructions to the candidate match the instructions to the examiners
- Examiners must be thoroughly briefed on the station
- Examiners must be given sufficient time to review materials such as the instructions for the candidate, marking schemes, and the findings of the SPs
- Examiners should actively take part during the pilot testing of the stations

Next, we present an example of instructions to the examiner. We will use the previous example of Madam Sufia, who suffers from generalized anxiety disorder.

Below is an example of instructions to the examiners.

This station will assess the candidate's ability to

- Obtain a focused history of a patient with generalized anxiety disorder
- Use verbal and nonverbal communication effectively in a medical set-up

Expected level of competency

- Obtain a focused history of generalized anxiety disorder
- Demonstrate verbal and nonverbal communication appropriately

Important information

- Your role is to observe and mark the candidate according to the marking template
- A standardized patient (SP) will portray the role of the patient
- You will only observe the candidate interacting with the SP
- You are not allowed to ask questions or provide comments or feedback to the candidate during the examination
- Please write brief comments about the candidate's clinical skills

Background information of the patient

- Name: Madam Sufia
- Age: 25 years
- Marital status: Single
- Education: University graduate
- Employment: Office administrator
- Language: Bilingual, able to communicate in English
- Premorbid condition: None
- Current medication: None
- Associated medical/surgical condition: None
- Set-up: General practitioner's office

Description of the problem

Madam Sufia has been suffering from intense fear whenever she comes near an elevator. This has been going on for the last 3 years. However, the fear has been getting more intense during the last couple of months.

(Continued)

(*Continued*)

Characteristics of attacks

- Breathing difficulty
- Palpitations
- Choking sensation
- Trembling of hands
- Sweating; especially on palms and soles
- Feeling of throwing up

The attacks are not associated with hearing strange voices or seeing visions. Nobody tries to manipulate her thoughts or behaviors. She cannot remember any specific event that led to this anxiety. She does not have any significant childhood mental trauma or abuse.

She does not have any suicidal thoughts. She has no history of depression. No other family member has similar symptoms.

Preparing Equipment and Materials

The station developers should also prepare and submit a list of equipment and materials that are needed for the station in a standard format. Increasingly, mannequins and simulation devices are used in OSCEs. Although it is the role of the administrators and technicians to set-up the simulators and mannequins, it is the responsibility of the station developers to verify the findings and ensure that the devices are in proper working order. It is useful to instruct the examiners on the basic mechanisms and troubleshooting of the devices. It is recommended that there should be spare mannequins or simulators with technicians available during the OSCE. Examiners and station developers should be vigilant for common mistakes, such as:

- Malfunction/unavailability of the power sources or battery;
- Change of set-ups of the mannequins during the examination;
- Failure to remove the key to the condition in the simulator.

Once the OSCE Central Committee receives requisition lists for all OSCE stations, a master list needs to be created for the entire examination. A master list might look like this (Table 6.1):

Table 6.1. Example of a Master List for Equipment and Materials

Station	Simulated/ Standardized Patient	Examiner	Materials/ Equipment	Comments
Hand hygiene	None	1 (staff nurse)	Chlorhexidine hand-rub: 2 sets	—
Gowning	None	1 (staff nurse)	Disposable gowns, garbage disposal, face masks, sterile gloves	Keep extra materials
Developmental assessment	Mother and child	1	Toys, tools for development assessment, milk/formula, diapers	1 extra pair of mother and child for each round
Cardiovascular examination	None	1	Harvey mannequins; hand-wash; Harvey's stethoscope	Cover-up Harvey's key to the conditions
Communication	1 (male)	1	Bottled water	Middle-aged male; native language speaker

In addition to station-specific requirements, certain equipment and materials are generally needed for the entire examination. Below is a sample list of equipment and materials that are needed during an OSCE:

- Stop watch
- Bell
- Pencils
- Erasers
- Laptops
- Glue tag
- Refreshments
- Thermometer
- Stethoscope

In addition to the above physical resources, some human resources are also needed centrally to run an OSCE effectively. These include a time keeper and marshals to direct traffic and trouble-shoot where necessary. Certain stations that require extensive reconfiguration of the station equipment after each candidate may need a dedicated station attendant. For example, a station that requires the candidate to set up a saline drip on a simulated upper limb may require a station attendant to remove the drip set from the limb and reposition all of the equipment at the end of each candidate's attempt. It is also imperative to have strict guidelines in order to safeguard against a breach in examination security.

Ensuring examination security

- All SPs, examiners, and others who have access to examination materials must sign a confidentiality agreement
- No-one is allowed to take instruction sheets back with them
- Conduct station-specific briefings for examiners, SPs, and administrators in order to protect the security of the entire examination
- Do not share examination blueprints with SPs in advance
- Information must be shared only on a need-to-know basis

Summary

The success of an OSCE depends on many inter-related components. Each component acts like a link in a chain. The strength of the chain depends on the strengths of each individual link. If a link of a chain is weak, the entire chain is weakened. Instructions to the candidates, instructions to the examiners, and instructions to the standardized patients or simulated patients need to be carefully reviewed in order to ensure consistency among the three sets of instructions. OSCE station writers and OSCE administrators should work together to prepare station-specific checklists in order to minimize the chances of errors.

References

Adamo G. (2003) Simulated and standardized patients in OSCEs: Achievements and challenges 1992–2003. *Med Teach* **25**(3): 262–270.

Amin Z, Chong YS, Khoo HE. (2006) *Practical Guide to Medical Student Assessment*, 1st ed. World Scientific Publishing, Singapore.

Cleland JA, Abe K, Rethan J-J. (2009) The use of simulated patients in medical education: AMEE Guide No. 42. *Med Teach* **31**(6): 477–486.

Selby C, Osman L, Davis M, Lee M. (1995) How to do it: Set up and run an objective structured clinical exam. *Br Med J* **310**(6988): 1187–1190.

van der Vleuten CPM, Swanson DB. (1990) Assessment of clinical skills with standardized patients: State of the art. *Teach Learn Med* **2**(2): 58–76.

7

CREATING A SCORING TEMPLATE FOR ASSIGNING MARKS

Scoring or marking template captures the candidate's competence level as judged by the examiners during an OSCE. As such, it is one of the most critical of the elements that determine the success of the OSCE. It has a considerable impact on the validity, reliability, and educational impact of the OSCE. It is our observation that scoring templates of OSCEs in many places are either poorly constructed or faulty. Therefore, we provide a comprehensive coverage on the topic.

At the end of this chapter, we should be able to:

(i) Critically review the pros and cons of different types of scoring template.
(ii) Discuss the features of itemized checklists and global ratings.
(iii) Compare global ratings with itemized checklists.
(iv) Develop a fit-for-purpose scoring template for a given OSCE.

☝ Good to Know

Some authors make a distinction between scoring and marking. Strictly speaking, scoring refers to live assignment of marks while the OSCE is in progress and marking refers to the process that takes place after the OSCE is over. In this book, for the purposes of simplicity, we make no distinction between scoring and marking.

Purpose of a Scoring Template

The primary purpose of a scoring template is to capture the candidate's actions and interactions during the OSCE. A scoring template contains all of the important tasks that the candidate is supposed to complete while at an OSCE station complete with the marks assigned for each task. Fundamentally, a scoring template contains either an itemized checklist (Fig. 7.1) or a global rating (Fig. 7.6).

A scoring template is not just a sheet of paper for the assignment of marks to the candidate. During an OSCE, the scoring template captures many facets of interactions and other valuable information that serve important functions:

- Quality assurance: A scoring template allows systematic data collection of the cohort's performance for a given OSCE station. A good scoring template coupled with systematic post-examination reviews identifies potential strengths and weaknesses in the curriculum or students' clinical experience, which should then be conveyed to the curriculum team for future actions. In addition, such reviews provide information that can be used to evaluate the station.
- Feedback: An itemized, checklist-based scoring template collects examiners' observations about the candidate's performance during the examination. Therefore, it is very useful for providing targeted and objective feedback to the candidate.
- Standard settings: A scoring template using a global rating may be used for setting the standard (i.e. pass/fail boundary) in the examination — a topic that will be dealt with in greater detail in Chapter 9.

Different Formats of Itemized Checklists

Itemized checklists are used for simplifying data collection during the examination, with the intention of improving objectivity and therefore the reliability of the examination. An itemized checklist includes all of the necessary observable tasks that the candidates are

Station: Examination of the chest		
Instruction to the examiner: Please check all the boxes that are applicable		
Introduces self	1	0
Asks for permission before proceeding to exam	1	0
Uses hand-rub before touching the patients	1	0
Assesses for symmetry of chest rise	1	0
Assesses for adequate chest movements	1	0
Counts the respiratory rate	1	0
Palpates for tracheal deviation	1	0
Auscultates for breath sounds (front)	1	0
Auscultates for breath sounds (axilla)	1	0
Auscultates for breath sounds (back)	1	0
Percusses the chest (axilla)	1	0
Percusses the chest (front)	1	0
Percusses the back (with hand folded in front)	1	0
Checks for vocal fremitus	1	0
Good sequence	1	0
Correct technique	1	0
Uses hand-rub after the examination	1	0
Courteous throughout	1	0

1= Performed; 0= Not performed

Fig. 7.1. An simplified itemized checklist; binary scoring (1 and 0) restricts the examiner's ability to mark a candidate on a graded scale.

expected to demonstrate in that given station (Gorter *et al.*, 2000). The nature and extent of the checklist depends on the tasks to be performed during the OSCE and may vary from a simple "yes/no" format to more elaborate ones with greater ability to capture a candidate's competence as a range (i.e. on a graded scale). Fig. 7.1

depicts a simplified itemized checklist for chest examination for preclinical students.

Let us critically review the features of this checklist (Fig. 7.1):

- It is simple, being easy to complete by an examiner;
- It is objective and less prone to marking variations between the examiners;
- All items, both the important and not-so-important ones, carry equal marks;
- It is process driven; the candidate only needs to perform the steps to get the marks.

However, there are several significant shortcomings with this checklist (Reznick *et al.*, 1998):

- This checklist does not capture the candidate's ability to *elicit or interpret* the findings;
- If pathological findings are present, there has to be an avenue to capture the candidate's findings either in writing or through discussion. This checklist does not provide such an opportunity;
- There is no gradation of marks for partial performance of a task. For example, suppose a candidate has performed percussion; however, the technique is unsatisfactory. There is no scope for the examiner to assign a partial mark to the candidate;
- All of the items carry equal marks; therefore, it is possible to score highly at this station without even performing some of the critical steps. For example, a candidate might not perform auscultation, which is critical in chest examination, and still can get a very high mark;
- There is no scope for the examiner to fail or give extra credit to the candidate for elements of competencies that are not listed in the checklist. For example, if a candidate follows the steps listed in the checklist but is very crude during the process of the clinical examination, the checklist does not permit the examiner to penalize the candidate for undesirable behaviors;
- A candidate might not carry out all of the steps in the order that is listed. For example, a candidate may auscultate the chest before percussing. There are no instructions to the examiner within this marking template for such a situation.

It is our observation that many checklists in OSCEs are similar to this checklist (Fig. 7.1). While this type of checklist does have some value in the early clinical years when the focus of the examination is to ascertain the candidate's ability to carry out basic examination techniques in a standardized manner, these are oversimplified and unable to capture the richness, complexity, and variability of clinical encounters. For the clinical years, checklists need to be much more sophisticated, with an emphasis on the interpretation and clinical application of data generated through history taking or physical examination.

How can we overcome the problems depicted above without compromising the objectivity and reliability of the OSCE? Several modifications can be made to improve the scoring template:

- Graded marking schemes allow examiners to award differential marks based on the candidate's performance;
- Assigning higher marks for items that are critical for the task and relatively lower marks for items that are not so critical;
- Creating an avenue for the candidate to present their findings either verbally or in writing;
- Allocating additional marking for overall performance during the examination;
- Introducing global marking with good anchors.

Let us contrast the checklist depicted in Fig. 7.1 with the following example (Fig. 7.2). This is also a chest examination station. The candidate's task is to perform a chest examination and interpret the findings. Assume the content experts (i.e. the clinicians) have identified percussion and auscultation as two critical components of the process. Note that much higher marks have been assigned to these two critical components as compared with other less essential ones. It is unlikely that a candidate would pass the station if he/she fails to perform auscultation and percussion properly. Examiners can also provide marking in a graded manner — full marks for carrying out a task properly, half marks for carrying out a task with some deficiencies, and no marks for not carrying out the task or doing it poorly.

Station: Examination of the chest			
Preliminaries (maximum 1.5 marks)			
Introduces self		0.5	0
Requests for permission before proceeding to examine		0.5	0
Uses hand-rub before touching the patient		0.5	0
Inspection (maximum 3 marks)			
Assesses for symmetry of chest rise		1	0
Assesses for adequate chest movement		1	0
Counts the respiratory rate		1	0
Palpation (maximum 2 marks)			
Palpates for tracheal deviation		1	0
Checks for vocal fremitus		1	0
Auscultation (maximum 6 marks)			
Auscultates the front	2	1	0
Auscultates the axilla	2	1	0
Auscultates the back (with hand folded in front)	2	1	0
Percussion (maximum 6 marks)			
Percusses the front	2	1	0
Percusses the axilla	2	1	0
Percusses the back (with hand folded in front)	2	1	0
Closure (maximum 1.5 mark)			
Thanks the patient		0.5	0
Uses hand-rub after touching the patient		1	0

2= Does well; 1= Completed, but with some deficiencies; 0 = Did not carry out or did poorly

Fig. 7.2. A modified version of the checklist with greater marking assigned to critical components of the tasks.

Too much objectivity and rigidity in the marking template may compromise the usefulness of the OSCE. A high degree of objectivity may interfere with the validity of the examination and may promote rote repetition of steps in clinical examination without interpretation and application.

The above marking template can be further modified to include the presentation and interpretation of findings and overall competency during the examination (Fig. 7.3). Note that in this checklist, 6 marks (30% of the total) are assigned to percussion and auscultation. Another 6 marks (30% of the total) are assigned to interpretation

Station: Examination of the chest				
Preliminaries (maximum 1 mark)	1	0.5	0	
Inspection (maximum 2 marks)	2	1	0	
Palpation (maximum 2 marks) Palpates for tracheal deviation Checks for vocal fremitus	1 1	0 0		
Auscultation (maximum 3 marks)	3	2	1	0
Percussion (maximum 3 marks)	3	2	1	0
Closure (maximum 1 mark)	1	0.5	0	
Overall impression (maximum 2 marks)	2	1	0	
Presentation of findings (maximum 3 marks)	3	2	1	0
Arriving at correct diagnosis (maximum 3 marks)	3	2	1	0

Fig. 7.3. A checklist that captures the interpretation of patient findings and a candidate's ability to arrive at a diagnosis.

and diagnosis. It is unlikely that the candidate would pass this station without having completed these tasks competently.

There are several ways that the last two items in the checklist (presentation of findings and arriving at a correct diagnosis) can be captured:

(i) Presentation to the examiner, or;
(ii) Write down the findings and diagnosis as a closed response or in a free text format (see below), or;
(iii) Having a separate linked station (discussed in Chapter 5) where the findings and the correct diagnosis can be supplemented by additional competencies, such as interpretation of X-rays, explanation of findings to the patient, or formulating a management option.

These formats (Figs. 7.2 and 7.3) of scoring template have several advantages over the rigid marking template depicted in Fig. 7.1:

• The scoring template captures tasks that are germane to the station; hence, it has greater authenticity and higher validity;

- Examiners have greater flexibility to mark the candidate according to their level of performance. For example, a candidate who auscultated before percussing can be penalized using the individual ratings as well as the global rating (i.e. overall impression of the examiner regarding the candidate);
- It gives a higher weighting to the items that are important; therefore, a candidate who is unable to perform these crucial steps correctly is likely to justifiably fail the station.

However, greater flexibility in marking may also lead to lower objectivity. As the examiners are given more leeway to use their judgment, it is crucial that the examiners are thoroughly briefed on the competency to be expected and standardize their marking through detailed discussion. Prior cohort data, simulated videos demonstrating the different levels of competence, and a review of captured videos of previous examinations may help the examiners to standardize their marking.

The scoring template depicted in Fig. 7.2 is still process oriented; that is, this template does not capture the candidate's ability to detect abnormal and normal findings and diagnose a condition from these findings. If the focus of the station includes these competencies, we have to allow the candidate to write down their findings and their diagnosis. Alternatively, they can express their findings verbally to the examiner. The candidate can write down their findings either as a closed-ended or a free text response. A combination of closed-ended and free text responses is also possible. Assume that the patient (i.e. the mannequin) has a right-sided pneumothorax. Figure 7.4 presents an example of how we can capture the information in this case. Note that the space for the diagnosis is intentionally provided as a free text format in order to prevent the candidate from deriving a clue about the possible findings.

Qualitative Comments

Marking templates are, in general, quantitative in nature; marks are assigned in a numeric format. It might be useful to have a provision

```
The trachea is (choose one response)
       □ Centrally located
       □ Deviated to the left
       □ Deviated to the right

Percussion note (choose one response)
       □ Normal on both sides
       □ Hyper-resonant on the right
       □ Dull on the right
       □ Hyper-resonant on the left
       □ Dull on the left

Auscultation (choose one response)
       □ Normal on both sides
       □ Diminished on the right
       □ Diminished on the left

Write down the most likely diagnosis in the space provided:
```

Fig. 7.4.   Example of a scoring sheet for capturing a candidate's response.

for the examiners to write qualitative comments about a candidate's performance during a given OSCE. Such qualitative comments capture the on-the-spot impressions of the expert examiners. Qualitative comments are also very useful in potentially contentious situations, such as when a candidate fails or receives exceptionally high marks.

Generic Marking Template

So far, we have discussed scoring templates that are very specific to a given station. This means that each station, even when the station is related to the same body system or competency, needs a separate marking template. However, in certain situations, it might be possible to use a generic marking template for several related stations. A generic marking template is used in multi-station clinical examinations, such as PACES examination in the Membership of the Royal College of Physicians, UK (web address: http://www. mrcpuk.org/paces/pages/pacesmarksheets.aspx). A generic marking template specifies the competency expected for each domain in general terms (Fig. 7.5).

Recommended practice for itemized checklist construction

- Link the items under the checklist with the station objectives
  - o Rationale: To capture important tasks
- Keep an itemized checklist-based scoring template for tasks that are specific
  - o Rationale: Tasks that are more generic (e.g. communication skills) may be better captured with global rating scales
- Keep the items in the checklist to a manageable 10–12 items (Vu *et al.*, 1992)
  - o Rationale: To reduce cognitive load on the examiners and to improve the accuracy of the data captured
- Provide greater weighting to items that are critical to the tasks
  - o Rationale: To ensure that the candidates do not pass without carrying out the critical tasks adequately
- Ensure that each item in the checklist captures related aspects of the tasks; e.g. inspection, palpation, auscultation, and percussion of abdomen should be kept as separate items instead of grouping them together
  - o Rationale: To ensure greater objectivity of the data collection
- Allocate marks for interpretations of findings and their implications on management
  - o Rationale: To capture clinical reasoning and management by the candidate
- Where necessary, provide the examiner with the opportunity to grade the behavior of the candidate through a simplified rating scale
  - o Rationale: To enable differentially rewarding the excellent candidates and thereby enhancing the discriminatory power of the station
- Include items that not only address technical skills but also the soft skills; e.g. communication skills, empathy, and professionalism
  - o Rationale: To develop integrated stations that better reflect and simulate real-life performance

(*Continued*)

(*Continued*)

- Encourage examiners to provide qualitative comments, especially for candidates performing poorly
  - o Rationale: Enable objective feedback to the candidate
- Peer-review and pilot the checklist before using it for summative purposes
  - o Rationale: It is crucial to establish that the checklist can be implemented within the allotted time, that it captures the essential behavior of the candidate, and that it is interpreted similarly by different examiners

The generic marking template reduces the workload related to developing an itemized marking sheet. However, as the generic marking template is based on experts' judgments, successful implementation depends on rigorous moderation exercises among the examiners in order to determine the expected levels of competence. It is also essential that such a generic template has a set of descriptors anchoring either all of the rating points or at least some of the rating points, as shown in Fig. 7.5.

Global Rating

"Ironically, the strengths of the checklists may be its biggest weakness: many critics feel that checklists in general reward thoroughness rather than competence and penalize efficiency."

Reznick *et al.* (1998)

Global rating is an *overall judgment* of the candidate's competence during the examination. It is an impression that an expert examiner or observer develops after observing the candidate's performance during the OSCE. An example of a typical global rating is shown in Fig. 7.6:

Domains	Good	Satisfactory	Poor
History taking	Systematic and thorough		Disorganized, partial
	Elicits history related to major presenting problem		Fails to address major presenting problem
	Includes past medical, surgical, family, and drug history		Does not include past medical, surgical, family, and drug history
	Takes psychosocial and financial history		Does not take psychosocial and financial history
	Assesses impact of the illness on patient and family		Does not assess impact of illness
Physical examination	Systematic		Haphazard
	Maintains patient comfort throughout		Makes patient uncomfortable
	Fluent and efficient		Disorganized
	Correct technique		Incorrect technique
Differential diagnoses (D/D)	Sensible D/D		Irrelevant D/D
	Prioritizes the D/D		No priority
	Includes key diagnosis		Does not include key diagnosis
	No implausible diagnosis		Implausible diagnosis
Management	Coherent and practical		Incoherent and impractical
	Appropriate to the conditions		Inappropriate or incorrect
	Considers socioeconomic factors		No consideration given for socioeconomic factors
	Considers patient/family preferences		
	Includes management of complications		Management plan is nonspecific to the patient
Communication	Uses nonverbal and verbal communication		Poor use of verbal and non-verbal communication
	Appropriate use of open-ended and closed-ended questions		Predominantly closed-ended questions
	Treats patient with dignity and respect		Abrupt or rude
	Upholds patient safety		Undermines patient safety

Fig. 7.5. A generic marking template used in a multi-station clinical examination.

Excellent	Good	Satisfactory	Borderline	Fail

Fig. 7.6. A global rating template.

Debate is ongoing whether global rating is better than or equivalent to itemized marking templates and their relative merits (Cunnington, Neville, & Norman, 1997). Longer checklists tend to undermine the wholeness of the tasks by deconstructing the tasks into multiple mini-tasks and so reward thoroughness rather than efficiency (Hodges *et al.*, 1999). Some notable studies (Hodges *et al.*, 1999; Regehr *et al.*, 1998) identified global rating as superior to or as good as itemized marking templates. Global rating, if done properly by expert examiners, may be able to achieve higher levels of consistency in marking (Regehr *et al.*, 1998).

Let us compare and contrast itemized marking and global rating templates. Itemized marking allows greater objectivity and structured feedback to be given to the candidate. It also requires less rigorous faculty training as compared with an OSCE with only global ratings. However, global rating templates:

- Provide a more holistic interpretation of a candidate's competency and capture aspects of competencies that are not typically captured by itemized marking;
- Are more open to subjective interpretation, and hence need careful calibration by the experts;
- May not indicate the underlying reasoning of the examiners when they assign a particular mark to the candidate (Dauphinee *et al.*, 1997);
- May capture elements of physician competencies that are not captured by itemized marking;
- May be more appropriate than an itemized checklist for physicians' tasks that are more generic in nature, such as counseling and communication, or tasks that are complex in nature, such as patient management.

Other uses of global rating are to:

(i) Set standards for the OSCE using the borderline group or the borderline regression method (see Chapter 9);
(ii) Reward or penalize candidates on aspects of competencies that are not captured by itemized marking;

(iii) Provide the opportunity for the examiner to supplement the checklist with his/her holistic judgment.

The itemized marking templates is more suitable for:

- Clinical tasks that are highly standardized, such as cardiopulmonary resuscitation;
- Procedural skills;
- Early clinical years when the candidate is learning a clinical task.

Global rating is more suitable for:

- Generic skills, such as communication and counseling;
- When the station objective is the assessment of clinical judgment;
- Patient management.

It is our recommendation to use, in most cases, both itemized marking as well as global rating templates in order to take advantages of both formats.

Summary

The scoring template is one of the most important elements of an OSCE station. Sadly, mistakes in the development of marking templates are common. The itemized marking template, which is a good method for improving objectivity, needs to be developed in such a way that the tasks that are captured in the checklist do not become too mechanistic and reductionist. Wherever appropriate, scoring templates should be designed to capture data interpretation, application of knowledge, clinical management, clinical judgment, and humanistic aspects of medicine, in addition to carrying out the tasks. The global rating template, which is a more subjective interpretation of candidate performance by the examiners, requires more examiner training and greater consensus among the examiners on the expected level of competence.

References

Cunnington JPW, Neville AJ, Norman GR. (1997) The risks of thoroughness: Reliability and validity of global ratings and checklist in an OSCE. In: Scherpbier AJJA, van der Vleuten CPM, Rethans JJ, van der Steed AFW (eds). *Advances in Medical Education*. Kluwer, The Netherlands, pp. 143–145.

Dauphinee WD, Blackmore DE, Smee S, Rothman AI, Reznick R. (1997) Using the judgments of physician examiners in setting the standards for a national multi-center high stakes OSCE. *Adv Health Sci Educ* 2(3): 201–211.

Gorter S, Rethan JJ, Scherpbier A, van der Heijde D, Houben H, van der Vleuten, van der Linden S. (2000) Developing case-specific checklist for standardized-patient-based assessments in internal medicine: A review of literature. *Acad Med* 75(11): 1130–1137.

Hodges B, Regehr G, McNaughton N, Tiberius R, Hanson M. (1999) OSCE checklists do not capture increasing levels of expertise. *Acad Med* 74(10): 1129–1134.

Regehr, G, MacRae H, Reznick RK, Szalay D. (1998) Comparing the psychometric properties of checklists and global rating scales for assessing performance on an OSCE-format examination. *Acad Med* 73(9): 993–997.

Reznick R, Regehr G, Yee G, Rothman A, Blackmore D, Dauphinee D. (1998) Process rating forms versus task specific checklists in an OSCE for medical licensure. *Acad Med* 73(10 suppl): S97–S99.

Vu NV, Marcy MM, Colliver JA, Verhulst SJ, Travis TA, Barrows HS. (1992) Standardized (simulated) patients' accuracy in recording clinical performance check-list items. *Med Educ* 26(2): 99–104.

8

PREPARING PATIENTS FOR THE OSCE

When the OSCE was first introduced about four decades ago, real patients were very much part and parcel of the OSCE (Collins & Harden, 1998). Then, however, Howard Barrows introduced programmed patients (Barrows & Abrahamson, 1964) into clinical assessment in order to reduce the variability in the patient presentation at the examination. Programmed patients later included both standardized patients (real patients or lay persons, coached to deliver a standard act) and simulated patients (coached lay persons) for training and assessment. We recommend, in most instances, that simulated patients to be standardized patients.

At the end of this chapter, we should be able to:

(i) Recognize that patients used in the OSCE come with a range of possibilities.
(ii) Determine the pros and cons of standardized and simulated patients in an OSCE.
(iii) Make an educated choice between standardized patients, simulated patients, and simulators in a high-stake OSCE.

The nature of patients or materials to be used in the examination may vary from real patients, standardized patients, simulated patients, mannequins and task trainers, audiovisual materials, or a combination of these. Real patients in an authentic work environment may be used to assess physicians' on-the-job performance (Ponnamperuma, 2013; Wass *et al.*, 2001). The tools used for this purpose include the mini-Clinical Evaluation Exercise (mini-CEX), Direct Observations of Procedural Skills (DOPS), or other tools that measure performance at the "Does" level of Miller's pyramid (Ponnamperuma, 2013). These encounters do not take place in examination situations and hence are out of the scope of this discussion. The use of materials — mostly simulators, mannequins, and related technologies — in an OSCE will be discussed in the next chapter. The focus of this chapter is to discuss issues pertaining to the use of standardized and simulated patients in the setting of an OSCE.

👆 Good to Know

"SP", the commonly used abbreviation in the context of an OSCE, has a dual meaning. SP may mean "standardized patient" or "simulated patient". Although these two terms are used interchangeably, it is important to ensure that any patient, real or simulated, used in the examination needs to have some degree of standardization.

In this book, we have primarily used the term "simulated patient" to denote a trained volunteer who acts as a patient, whereas the term "standardized patient" is used to denote a real or simulated patient who has been coached to reproduce histories and/or physical signs consistently across all candidates.

How we decide whether to use standardized patients, simulated patients, or mannequins and task trainers in an OSCE depends on several inter-related factors:

(i)   The relative balance between standardization and maintaining the authenticity of the task;
(ii) The degree of realism expected from the patients or patient substitutes;
(iii) The nature of the tasks tested in the examination;
(iv) The purpose of the OSCE;
(v)   The logistics and practical considerations.

Balance between Standardization and Authenticity

The very term "OSCE" suggests that a certain degree of standardization is an explicit agenda of the examination. Attempts to standardize examination-related variables, especially patients and examiners, to the extent possible without compromising the nature of the task, should be a core feature of any OSCE. However, attempts to mimic a real clinical environment through having more authentic examination materials might undermine the standardization, as the clinical environment is inherently variable and complex

☝ Good to Know

Standardization: Variability in the examination may result from several sources, including patients, examiners, and examinees. Of course, examinees' variability is related to the competence of the examinee in the examination and is the primary point of interest in the examination. A fair and credible examination attempts to minimize variability or sources of errors related to patients and examiners. Patients, whether real or actors, are "standardized" so that they portray findings or provide information in a fairly uniform manner during the entire examination. Examiners are provided with training, clear instructions, and scoring sheets to reduce variability in order to improve standardization during the examination. Generally speaking, higher standardization leads to better reliability by reducing unintended variability in the examination.

Authenticity: Authenticity, in the context of clinical examination, refers to the degree to which the examination faithfully replicates the natural practice environment. In an ideal environment, the tasks that the examinees are supposed to perform and examination materials (patients, mannequins, etc.) should resemble the real clinical practice environment. For logistical and other reasons, it might not be possible to achieve this in every situation. Therefore, alternatives such as mannequins or standardized or simulated patients are used. Generally speaking, higher authenticity in the clinical examination results in greater validity, as every clinical examination strives to replicate the clinical environment.

in nature (Bokken *et al.*, 2008). The tension between standardization and replicating the clinical environment while preserving authenticity deserves further discussion.

While standardization of the examination is a desirable goal, over-standardization might actually undermine the validity of the examination (Kneebone *et al.*, 2007; Kneebone, 2009). Strategies to increase standardization in clinical examinations are directed either towards manipulating the scoring template, patients, or patient substitutes (e.g. simulated patients, mannequins, or audio-visual materials). In Chapter 7, we presented in detail the perils of scoring templates that incorporate a long list of checklist items. We have learned that such a long, static checklist may unjustifiably compromise the efficiency of data gathering and hence may not reflect the practice of experts (Hodges *et al.*, 1999). In such a situation, expert or consultants may score lower in the OSCE than novices (i.e. junior residents).

Real or simulated patients are standardized to a certain degree in the way they provide their history, communicate with examinees, or portray physical findings. Over-standardization in this context might jeopardize the validity of the examination by not faithfully replicating the complexity and variability inherent in patients in real-life. Trainees may get used to classical, textbook descriptions of a patient's problem, and may have difficulty in dealing with real patients with variable findings.

Degree of Realism as Portrayed by the Patients

Real patients in an examination can be used with varying degrees of reality and imposed standardization. Therefore, it is more accurate to depict the degree of reality that is portrayed by the real patients in clinical examinations on a continuous scale rather than with a simple "yes" or "no." At one extreme, although this is not recommended, a real patient might be included in the examination without any prior briefing (Collins & Harden, 1998; Ponnamperuma *et al.*, 2009). More reasonably, real patients can be coached and

Table 8.1. Examples of Different Types of Simulated and Real Patients

Range of Reality	Example
Uncoached real patients	A patient with metabolic syndrome is presented in the examination without training
Real patients portraying only certain physical findings	A patient with aortic regurgitation has incidental cataract; candidates are asked to examine relevant cardiovascular components only
Standardized patients trained to narrate only certain parts of their history	A patient with diabetes with asthma is coached to adhere only to the history of diabetes
Standardized patients that interact with candidates in a scripted manner	A thyrotoxicosis patient asks the candidates predetermined questions during the OSCE
Standardized patients that interact with candidates and respond to candidates' suggestions	A hypertensive patient asks the candidates questions and responds to the candidate's answers
Simulated patients trained to provide a history and interact with the candidate in a consistent manner	A trained volunteer acts as a patient with suicidal ideation in a station in order to assess the candidate's ability to determine suicide risk
Simulated patients trained to portray (i.e. mimic) physical findings	A trained volunteer portrays gait abnormality following a stroke

trained to provide histories, portray physical examinations, or communicate in a fairly uniform manner. Furthermore, depending on the context and tasks of the examination, real patients may or may not be expected to ask the examinees questions or interact proactively. Table 8.1 provides some examples in order to illustrate the different degrees of realism that can be provided by the patients in an examination.

Nature of Tasks to be Tested

Certain tasks that the examinees are expected to carry out during an OSCE inherently favor simulated patients or mannequins over real patients and vice versa (Bokken *et al.*, 2009). For example, emergency and acute situations, psychiatric conditions, and issues that are sensitive in nature are difficult to test in an examination using real patients. For these conditions, simulated patients, mannequins, or hybrid methods using both a simulated patient and a mannequin are preferable. If the task is technical in nature and a standard protocol exists, a mannequin or simulated patient is preferable over a real patient. If the tasks are invasive or intrusive in nature, it is almost mandatory that such stations require mannequins. The OSCE stations that primarily test communication and counseling skills may not need real patients. Finally, in the early part of clinical training, when there is a higher emphasis on skill acquisition rather than interpretation of investigations and patient management, simulated patients and mannequins should be sufficient.

Situations where simulated patients are preferable over real patients

- Patient education stations (e.g. behavior modifications)
- Communication stations (e.g. negotiations)
- History taking stations (e.g. headache)
- No abnormality is expected (e.g. normal eye examination)
- Focus is on the process of doing the task (e.g. performing abdominal examination in the preclinical years)
- Psychiatric conditions (e.g. anxiety disorders, suicide risk estimation, combative patients, etc)
- Sensitive issues (e.g. sexual history, alcoholism and substance abuse, abortion, obesity, etc)
- End-of-life discussion
- Breaking bad news (e.g. revealing cancer diagnosis)
- Medication errors/iatrogenic complications

(*Continued*)

(Continued)

- Intrusive examinations, such as per-rectal examination or breast examination (with a mannequin)
- Uncomfortable examinations, such as ophthalmoscopic examinations requiring pupillary dilatation (with a mannequin)
- Invasive procedures (e.g. venipuncture, lumbar puncture, venous cut down, etc)

Conversely, other tasks are inherently better suited for real patients who are standardized. For example, certain physical findings are difficult to portray, or the available mannequins portray the findings in a suboptimal manner. Alternatively, the portrayal could be unrealistically consistent or too far from reality. For example, it is difficult to faithfully produce findings such as an enlarged liver, edema, or joint abnormalities in rheumatological disorders in a mannequin or simulated patient. For these "fixed" physical findings, real patients with suitable findings are needed.

Examples of fixed physical findings where real patients are preferable

- Ascites
- Hepato-splenomegaly
- Joint swelling and abnormalities
- Dermatological conditions
- Lumps, lymph nodes, or goiters
- Edema
- Pregnancy
- Hyperthyroidism

Purpose of the OSCE

As the students and trainees progress through their training, there should be a gradual shift from skill acquisition (i.e. performing a task) to more value-added options, such as interpretation of clinical findings, deriving a diagnosis, proposing varying management options, and dealing with complex medical, social, and ethical issues. For these complex endeavours, real patients might be more appropriate, as dealing with complexities and uncertainties is an inherent part of clinical training. Similarly, in postgraduate examinations, incorporating real patients alongside simulated patients creates more challenging tasks that an advanced-level trainee should be expected to succeed at.

Logistics and Practical Considerations

Logistics and practical factors vary highly from one center to another. Logistical and practical factors that are important to consider include the availability of real patients or alternatives, the available of expertise in training simulated patients, and the availability of expert examiners, suitable venues, and ethical and medico–legal frameworks in the country. In some countries, real patients are more easily recruited and so it might be less costly to recruit and train real patients as compared with simulated patients. The inclusion of real patients, particularly when deployed in stations that test complex cognitive processes such as patient management, requires trained or expert clinicians as examiners. If out-of-hospital venues are to be used in order to implement the OSCE, only stable real patients can be used in the examination. Moreover, such out-of-hospital venues should be able to provide the first line of medical management should a patient suffer an emergency. Finally, the prevalent ethical or legal guidelines may limit recruitment of real patients in the examination.

Preparing Real Patients for the OSCE

Adherence to the Blueprint

The blueprint is an absolute requirement for a valid and credible examination, which has been discussed in greater detail in Chapter 4. The primary determining factor of whether to use a real

Relative advantages of using real, standardized patients in an OSCE

- Broadens the range and complexity of the tasks that can be tested in an OSCE
- Provides an opportunity to assess complex and challenging tasks
- Certain physical examination findings can only be assessed credibly using real patients
- When blended with simulated patients in an OSCE circuit, the use of real patients reduces the distinction between simulation and reality
- Real patients need less training and preparatory time as compared with lay persons used in the examination
- Real patients increase the credibility and acceptability of the examination for the students and examiners (Newble, 1991; Stillman *et al.*, 1990)

Relative disadvantages of using real patients in an OSCE

- May have higher variability and so reduce standardization
- Need for rigorous quality control, including blueprinting and faculty training
- Circuits may become dissimilar in terms of level of difficulty and types of patients to be examined
- Recruitment may be more troublesome and unpredictable as patients may fall sick on the day of examination

patient or alternatives in a given station should be the purpose of that particular station and the nature of the tasks to be performed during the examination. It might be that in a given OSCE, several real patients are needed. Conversely, the blueprint might dictate that in a given OSCE, there might not be any requirements for real patients. Therefore, adhering to the blueprint is of paramount importance. Under no circumstance should real patients be used just for the sake of having them in the examination or for reasons such as there being an interesting patient available on the ward!

Equivalency in Examination

It might be plausible that the pool of real patients recruited for the examination is not exactly similar. Even if a sufficient number of patients can be found with similar disease states, they might vary in their findings, extent and severity of diseases, and challenges posed to the examinees. For example, a station assessing a candidate's ability to diagnose a murmur may include several patients with different types of murmurs, such as aortic stenosis or mitral regurgitation. However, the Examination Committee should ensure that these patients, although they are not exactly the same, are equivalent in terms of the tasks to be performed on them and the level of difficulty represented by them.

Preparation of Case Summary

The Examination Committee must ensure that an adequate clinical summary is ready for every patient that is recruited for the examination well ahead of the scheduled examination. The case summary should include the pertinent history, findings, and preferred management options wherever relevant. Case summaries need to be vetted by the Examination Committee, who might recommend modifications to the case summary in order to fit the purposes of the examination.

Briefing of Patients

All real patients and their accompanying family members should be briefed about the examination. A general briefing targeting all patients should include the purpose and format of the examination, reporting requirements, schedule of the examination, and confidentiality agreement. More importantly, station-specific briefings should also be conducted. Station-specific briefings should include the tasks to be performed by the examinees, expected questions and answers, and the limits of the case. More elaborate practice sessions are recommended if the real patients are expected to interact with the examinees more meaningfully, such as asking questions, providing feedback, and grading. The briefing is an absolute necessity in order to increase the degree of standardization and objectivity of the OSCE.

Briefing of Examiners

The examiners' briefing is even more crucial for a successful OSCE with real patients, as the examiners are often content experts in their areas and they might have different expectations from the examinees. Moreover, examiners might vary in their interpretation of the clinical findings presented by the patient. The examiners' briefing aims to minimize the variability among the examiners. Station-specific briefings should specifically address the tasks to be performed during the examination, the clinical findings expected in the patients, key features of the case, the expected level of competency, and the marking criteria. If the examiners are to interact with examinees during the OSCE, suggested questions and acceptable answers should also be provided in writing.

Instructions to the Examinee

Like with all OSCE stations, the instructions to the examinee who is being assessed with real patients should be explicit. The instructions should include the tasks to be performed, whether the examinees are required to present their case summary to the examiners, and other specific information, such as whether asking for a history is unnecessary or whether there are any physical examinations that should not be performed on the patient.

Marking Template

The marking template for OSCE stations with real patients may take two different formats. If there is sufficient uniformity among the real patients for a given station, it might be possible to develop itemized marking templates, as in Fig. 7.3. Conversely, a generic marking template enabling greater subjective interpretations of the clinical findings, as in Fig. 7.5, may be used if the patients vary considerably in their findings.

Verification of Findings on the Day of Examination

It is imperative that the examiner(s) employed in a particular station verify the findings of the patients and match them against the case summary and marking template, because the patients' findings may change between the case write-up and the day of the examination.

Recruiting and Training Simulated Patients for the OSCE

As simulated patients are trained lay persons, but not necessarily professional actors, it is imperative that simulated patients are trained properly (Vu & Barrows, 1994). Before high-stakes summative examinations, the simulated patients' scenarios need to be piloted and the entire enactment needs to be validated by experts. In addition, the simulated patients might be required to mark the candidates during the OSCE.

The recruitment and training of simulated patients can be a very rewarding and enjoyable undertaking. With proper training, reward, and remuneration, simulated patients can be used for teaching, formative assessment, summative assessment, and feedback and remediation. Simulated patients can be recruited from a wide range of sources, including volunteers from the community, allied health professionals, students, and drama schools, among others. The aim should be to gradually expand the pool of simulated patients with continuous training, monitoring, and skills enhancement. Time permitting, newly recruited simulated patients could be given less intense roles, such as skills training and formative assessment, before progressing into higher-stakes examinations.

The training of simulated patients starts with a careful review of patient's condition, which may require an interview with real patients or a review of videos of a patient's condition. Simulated patients are

Review of case scenarios

⇩

Interview with simulated patients

⇩

Consultation with content specialists

⇩

Character preparation/make-up application/role-play

⇩

Pilot testing, feedback, and refinement

⇩

Rehearsing on the day of the OSCE

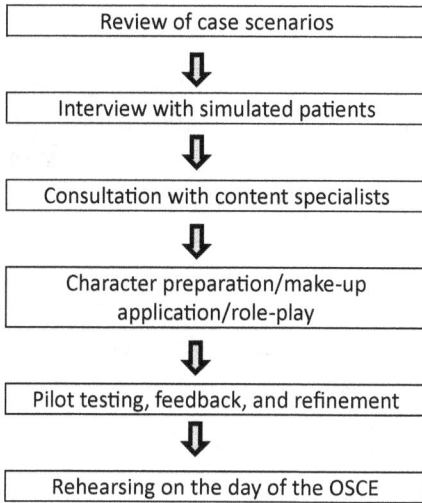

Fig. 8.1. Steps for recruiting and training a simulated patient.

then required to consult content experts and case writers in order to have a better insight into the case to be portrayed. Enactment of the case is carried out and pilot testing and practice runs are conducted. The depiction of the case may change at this point based on the feedback. Mannequins or simulators, if any, are then incorporated into the case. A live demonstration and practice run with an actual marking template are carried out during the examiners' briefing. We suggest that examiners take turns to be the candidate and interact with the simulated patient as in a real OSCE. At the same time, other examiners should observe the interaction and provide feedback to the simulated patient. We also strongly recommend rehearsing the enactment once again on the day of the OSCE.

There may be special instances where the simulated patients need the services of a make-up artist (e.g. to simulate a bruise, lump, etc). In such cases, careful planning is necessary in order to brief the make-up artist appropriately. In yet further instances, the simulated patients may need special training sessions in order to display clinical signs, such as accentuated reflexes or reduced air entry to one lung. These require specially trained trainers and simulated patients.

Summary

In summary, it is feasible and perfectly acceptable to have standardized real patients as well as simulated patients during an OSCE. The choice of which type of patient to use should be based on careful judgment of several inter-related factors, including the purpose of the given station, the degree of standardization and realism required, the nature of the tasks to be performed during the examination, and local logistical and practical considerations. Careful case selection, adherence to the examination blueprint, examiners' training, training of standardized and simulated patients, and a proper scoring template are crucial to the successful implementation of an OSCE, regardless of whether real or simulated patients are used in an OSCE.

References

Barrows HS, Abrahamson S. (1964) The programmed patient: A technique for apprising students' performance in clinical neurology. *J Med Educ* **39**: 802–805.

Bokken L, Rethans J-J, Scherpbier A, van der Vleuten CPM. (2008) Strengths and weaknesses of simulated and real patients in the teaching of skills to medical students: A review. *Simul Healthc* **3**(3): 161–169.

Bokken L, Rethans J-J, van Heurn, L Duvivier R, Scherpbier A, van der Vleuten CPM. (2009) Students' views on the use of real patients and simulated patients in undergraduate medical education. *Acad Med* **84**(7): 958–963.

Collins JP, Harden RM. (1998) AMEE Medical Education Guide No. 13: Real patients, simulated patients and simulators in clinical examinations. *Med Teach* **20**(6): 508–521.

Hodges B, Regehr G, McNaughton N, Tiberius R, Hanson M. (1999) OSCE checklists do not capture increasing levels of expertise. *Acad Med* **74**(10): 1129–1134.

Kneebone RL, Nestel D, Vincent C, Darzi A. (2007) Complexity, risk and simulation in learning procedural skills. *Med Educ* **41**(8): 808–814.

Kneebone R. (2009) Perspective: Simulation and transformational change: The paradox of expertise. *Acad Med* **84**(7): 954–957.

Newble DI. (1991) The observed long-case in clinical assessment. *Med Educ* **25**(5): 369–373.

Ponnamperuma G. (2013) Workplace based assessment. In: Walsh K (ed.), *Oxford Textbook of Medical Education*. Oxford University Press. UK, pp. 537–548.

Ponnamperuma GG, Karunathilake IM, McAleer S, Davis MH. (2009) The long case and its modifications: A literature review. *Med Educ* **43**(10): 936–941.

Stillman PL, Regan MB, Philbin M, Hayley HL. (1990) Results of a survey on the use of standardised patients to teach and evaluate clinical skills. *Acad Med* **65**(5): 288–292.

Vu NV, Barrows HS. (1994) Use of standardized patients in clinical assessments: Recent developments and measurement findings. *Educ Res* **23**: 23–30.

Wass V, van der Vleuten PCM, Shatzer J, Jones R. (2001) Assessment of clinical competence. *The Lancet* **357**(9260): 945–949.

9

PREPARING SIMULATORS FOR THE OSCE

In Chapter 8, we explored the use of standardized patients and simulated patients in the OSCE. We learned how standardized patients (trained real patients or lay persons) and simulated patients (lay persons) can emulate clinical scenarios during the OSCE to varying levels of realism. However, not all of the tasks and skills that are required for the assessment of clinical competency can be or should be tested on human beings — whether real patients or simulated patients. In this chapter, we will explore how the different types of simulators can broaden the domains of competency to be tested in the OSCE in a more objective manner and can complement the use of standardized and simulated patients in an OSCE.

At the end of this chapter, we should be able to:

(i) Describe various types of simulators that can enact realistic clinical scenarios;
(ii) Recognize how simulators and other relevant technological enhancements can broaden the range of skills to be tested in the OSCE;
(iii) Critically analyze the pros and cons of various types of simulators;
(iv) Incorporate the simulators and relevant technological innovations effectively into a summative OSCE.

👆 **Good to Know**

- Simulators: Machines and devices that emulate a clinical situation or a component of the human body. Examples include mannequins, anatomical models, computers, etc.
- Simulation: The process of recreating an authentic clinical scenario or clinical environment. It may or may not include the use of simulators. Examples include recreating a clinical scenario of a collapsed patient in the ward or testing the operative skills of a trainee.
- Hybrid simulation: In hybrid simulation, an assessor cleverly incorporates a simulator device into a human being in order to enhance realism. An example is attaching the breast task trainer to a simulated patient in order to test the candidate's ability to interact with the patient and conduct a physical examination of the breast simultaneously.

Simulators and Simulation in Medical Education

Primitive forms of simulators have been used for teaching for centuries in medicine. Physical models of the anatomy and diseases were constructed long before the advent of modern plastic models or computers (Cooper & Taqueti, 2004). Although the importance of deliberate practice in skill acquisition and maintenance has been known for quite some time, systematic and programmatic use of simulators and simulation in medical education had not been so successful in the past (Bradley, 2006). In recent years, the widespread availability of high-quality devices, the more favorable pricing of devices, and a general recognition of the importance of deliberate and repeated practice have provided much needed impetus towards the adoption of technology in medical education and assessment (Amin *et al.*, 2011; McGaghie *et al.*, 2006). The push for patient safety and a call for greater accountability and transparency have reinvigorated the discussion surrounding how we train and assess our students and trainees in critical life-saving skills. All of these developments have made the use of simulators and simulation in medical education a moral and ethical imperative (Dunn & Murphy, 2008; Ziv *et al.*, 2003).

The benefits of simulators and simulation have been widely recognized (Amin *et al.*, 2011; Cook *et al.*, 2011; Good, 2003; Issenberg *et al.*, 1999; Motola *et al.*, 2013). They offer the opportunity for developing individualized learning outcomes and learner-centric teaching and learning activities, promote an environment where mistake are forgiven, allow deliberate and repeated practice, and create an opportunity for feedback and reflection — all within a controlled and safe environment (Bradley, 2006; Motola *et al.*, 2013). The use of simulators has widened the horizons of the training and learning of health professionals by providing a portable, affordable, and efficient means to demonstrate how effective teaching and learning activities can lead to improvements in patient care. An increasing number of healthcare professionals-in-training have benefited from high-fidelity patient simulators in virtual hospitals (Brigden & Dangerfield, 2008). Clinical skills laboratories are no longer novelties, but now are part and parcel of the training and assessment protocols of nearly all developed healthcare teaching institutions (Bradley & Bligh, 2005). In recent years, more complex simulation scenarios have been implemented in health professionals' education. Examples of such highly sophisticated clinical scenarios include biodefense training exercises, wartime injury and preventive management training, aerial and high-speed trauma management simulation exercises, sports and occupational injury prevention and management, forensic evaluation, and learning complex surgical skills and interventional methods (Cooper & Taquety, 2004).

There are other notable advantages to using simulators in an OSCE. Simulators can reproduce a task in a standardized and consistent manner. The tasks can be repeated over and over again. Simulators also reduce the need for training standardized or simulated patients. Finally, in some countries, prevalent hospital policies or ethical standards may interfere with the recruitment of real patients for examination.

However, there are relative disadvantages to the use of simulators in an OSCE of which we should be aware. Not all clinical tasks can be tested using simulators. Even when a simulator or task

Table 9.1.   Relative Advantages and Disadvantages of Using Simulators in an OSCE

Advantages	Disadvantages
• Basic and difficult tasks/skills can be assessed in a safe and unthreatening environment	• Simulators are not suitable for all clinical tasks
• Any potentially harmful risk to patients is avoided	• The "textbook" or "prototypical" scenarios may not resemble real patients' findings
• Specific scenarios or tasks can be created easily	• Too much standardization may impede actual skill acquisition in real clinical settings
• Standardized checklists can be developed with relative ease	• May be costly to acquire and maintain
• Can be used with or without the involvement of an SP	• Need a well-equipped skills laboratory
• The tasks are reproducible over the entire examination period	• Candidates and examiners must be familiar with similar equipment

trainer is available, the level of reality that the simulators provide may not be adequate for the more advanced trainees. Finally, the fixed nature of clinical findings that a simulator typically provides may give trainees an impression that all patients with similar conditions will present in the same and consistent manner. For example, the unchanging and fixed nature of heart sounds that a simulator produces may lead the student to think that all real patients with similar heart conditions are to be expected to have the same auscultation findings. All of these advantages and disadvantages need to be considered within the context of the case scenario. Table 9.1 provides a summary of the relative advantages and disadvantages of using simulators in an OSCE.

Range of Simulators and Simulation

Simulators and simulation, along with standardized patients and simulated patients, provide a range of realism that can be effectively utilized during the OSCE. Although it is useful to view standard-ized patients, simulated patients, and simulators on a continuum (with real patients providing a higher degree of clinical authenticity and simulators providing a lower degree of clinical authenticity), in reality the spectrum of realism provided by simulators is also wide, with a considerable degree of overlap (Maran & Glavin, 2003). Moreover, in hybrid situations, both simulators and human beings are integrated within a given scenario.

Simplistically speaking, at one end there are low-fidelity simula-tors, such as anatomical models (e.g. breast or pelvis models) and task trainers (e.g. trainers for practicing suturing, chest tube insertion, or ophthalmological examination), while at the other end there are many sophisticated physiological mannequins that can respond to changes in stimuli (Lee, Grantham, & Boyd, 2008). For example, human patient simulators (HPSs) can portray blood pressure, oxygen saturation, and other physiological parameters in response to inter-ventions provided to the mannequins (Holcomb *et al.*, 2002). HPSs have been used extensively in cardiopulmonary resuscitation, trauma scenarios, and anesthesia team training (Holcomb *et al.*, 2002). Other examples of high-fidelity simulators include bron-choscopy and laparoscopy simulators that can track the skills of the candidate and provide a structured report at the end of the task. Somewhere in the middle of this spectrum are the simulators that do not respond to changes in stimuli, but are capable of producing realistic clinical findings, such as breath sounds and heart sounds. The Harvey® Cardiology Simulator is one such useful example (Sengupta *et al.*, 2007). Table 9.2 illustrates some of the examples of simulators that can be used in an OSCE.

Skills that can be Tested in the OSCE with Simulators

In the assessment of health professionals' education, simulators provide examiners with an opportunity to broaden the domains to be tested. A significant range of tasks can be tested using simula-tors, and for some tasks, there are no viable alternatives to using

Table 9.2.   Range of Simulators that can be Used in an OSCE

Anatomical models
- Pelvis
- Breast

Part task trainers
- Limb for suturing
- Ophthalmology (fundoscopy) trainer
- Ear examination trainer
- Male and female catheterization model
- Chest tube insertion trainer
- Intubation and airway mannequins

Physical examination skills (dynamic)
- Cardiac examination
- Breath sounds
- Abdominal examination

Virtual reality
- Bronchoscopy
- Laparoscopy
- Endoscopy

Physiological simulators
- Human patient simulators

Complex integrated simulators
- Virtual operating theater
- Virtual ward
- Virtual clinic
- Virtual trauma center

simulators (Winkel *et al.*, 2013). These include: infrequent but important clinical situations, such as responding to a collapsed patient; practical and procedural skills, such as chest tube insertion and suturing (Fig. 9.1); intrusive and intimate examinations that encroach upon patient privacy, such as per-vaginal or per-rectal examination (Fig. 9.2) (Hendrickx *et al.*, 2009); examinations that

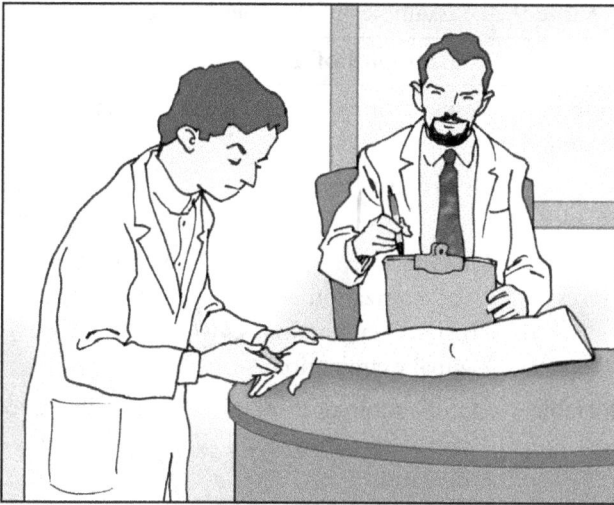

Fig. 9.1.   A simple task trainer can be used to test invasive procedures during an OSCE.

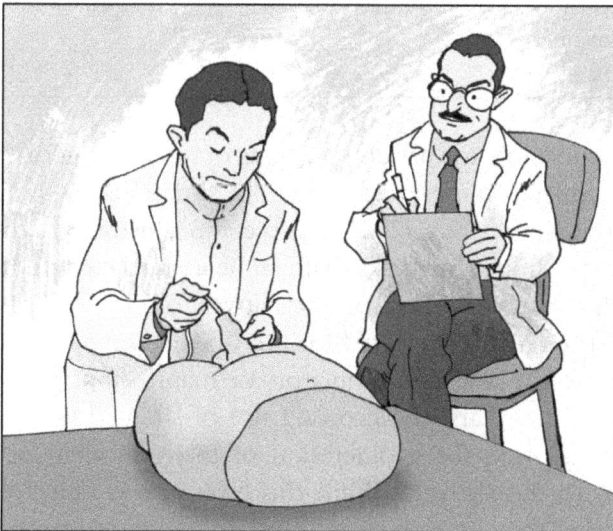

Fig. 9.2.   A mannequin in an OSCE for testing procedures that intrude on patients' privacy.

Table 9.3. Examples of Possible Uses of Simulators

Domain	Examples of Tasks	Simulator
Responding to an emergency	Resuscitation	SimMan® METI HPS®
Team performance	Obstructed labor	Hybrid simulation with labor trainer Noelle®
Intrusive procedures	Male/female catheterization Prostate examination Vaginal examination	Various mannequins Pelvic trainers
Uncomfortable tasks	Ophthalmological examination requiring pupil dilatation	Eye examination mannequins
Practical skills	Suturing and injections	Anatomical models or animal tissues
	Central line insertion	Task trainers
	Nasogastric tube insertion	Task trainers
Unsafe to perform on patients	Insulin injection	Anatomical models

are uncomfortable for patients, such as ophthalmological examination with dilated pupils; and teamwork situations, such as trauma code simulation (Amin, 2013). Table 9.3 illustrates some of the common but important tasks that can be easily tested in the OSCE for which there are no realistic alternatives to the use of simulators.

Once the tasks are selected for the OSCE, the next logical step is to choose the available simulators or mannequins for the given tasks. In recent years, the growing use of simulators and mannequins has allowed the proliferation of many models for medical educators to choose from. While this gives a wide range of option, it also makes the selection of appropriate simulators more difficult.

It is imperative that the choice of the simulator is based on the nature of the tasks that have been specified in the examination blueprint (see Chapter 4). The simulator should not be included in the examination just because it is available (Maran & Glavin, 2003).

Examples of different OSCE scenarios using simulators

Scenario 1

Task: A 45-year-old lady presents with a history of breast swelling for a few weeks. Take a focused history and examine the breast. Explain the examination findings to the patient.

Description: In this OSCE station, we can combine a standardized patient (SP) with the model for breast examination. The candidate will first interact with the patient to get a focused and appropriate history, and then he/she will perform the breast examination, the model for which is attached to the patient. The model had a swelling in the breast to simulate a breast cancer.

What is assessed? The candidate is assessed on history taking, clinical examination skills, and ability to make a provisional diagnosis.

Scenario 2

Task: A 65-year-old man presents with a history of urgency, hesitancy, and increased frequency of urination for a few months. Take a focused history from the patient and perform a per-rectal (PR) examination on the mannequin provided. Explain your findings to the attending examiner.

Description: In this case, we have also combined an SP with the model for PR examination. The candidate first interacts with the patient to obtain a focused and appropriate history, and then he/she performs the PR examination of the prostate on the model provided next to the patient. The model can simulate the different clinical features to be expected in common prostate pathologies.

What is assessed? The candidate is assessed on history taking, focused clinical examination skills, professionalism, and ability to make a provisional diagnosis.

Scenario 3

A 50-year-old patient presents with a history of urinary obstruction. Insert the Folly's catheter in order to evacuate the bladder on the model provided. Take usual aseptic precautions before you insert the catheter.

What is assessed? The candidate is assessed on the technical skills relevant to the early years of medical training; i.e. the ability of the candidate to insert the Folly's catheter into a patient in order to evacuate an obstructed urinary bladder.

Furthermore, for certain tasks, such as normal respiratory system examination and normal abdominal examination, the level of realism that the currently available simulators can provide may not be sufficient for the given level of training. In such cases, an alternative is to use a real human being (i.e. a simulated patient). Further, simulated patients could also be trained to illustrate not only normal findings, but also abnormal findings (e.g. an exaggerated knee jerk reflex, reduced air entry to one lung, etc).

Once we determine the right simulator that matches the tasks of the OSCE station, the next step is to develop the case scenario. The case scenario needs to be written for the use of the examination and the simulator needs to be prepared. The general guidelines for creating a scenario for an OSCE, as discussed in Chapter 6, are equally applicable to OSCE stations with simulators, with a few exceptions. Although there is no need for the training of standardized patients, it is imperative that the examiners are briefed on the basic functionality of the mannequins. There must be a technician available during the OSCE, especially for sophisticated mannequins. In a high-stakes summative OSCE, it is always recommended that a spare simulator is available in case of equipment malfunction.

Critical questions in selecting the right simulator

- Does the simulator match the assessment objectives/outcomes?
- Is the level of fidelity or the faithfulness of reproduction appropriate for the level of training and tasks?
- Are the students familiar with the simulator?
- Are the examiners familiar with the simulator?
- Do we have enough simulators, including a spare one, for the examination?
- Are there more easily available alternatives available for the task?

Summary

Simulators and related devices increase the breadth of clinical skills that can be tested during an OSCE. Simulators portray given clinical scenarios in a standardized and consistent manner. The range of simulators available has been increasing rapidly. The choice of a given simulator depends primarily on the objectives of the station. With a little bit of imagination and creativity, a simulator can be effectively integrated with a real human being in order to enhance the authenticity and realism of the case being portrayed.

References

Amin Z, Boulet JR, Cook DA, Ellaway R, Fahal A, Kneebone R, Maley M, Ostergaard D, Ponnamperuma G, Wearn A, Ziv A. (2011) Technology-enabled assessment of health professions education: Consensus statement and recommendations from the Ottawa 2010 conference. *Med Teach* **33**(5): 364–369.

Amin Z. (2013) Technology enhanced assessment in medical education. In: Walsh K (Ed.), *Oxford Textbook of Medical Education*. Oxford University Press, UK, pp. 489–499.

Bradley P. (2006) The history of simulation in medical education and possible future directions. *Med Educ* **40**(3): 254–262.

Brigden D, Dangerfield P. (2008) The role of simulation in medical education. *Clin Teach* **5**: 167–170.

Cook DA, Hatala R, Brydges R, Zendejas B, Szostek JH, Wang AT, Erwin P, Hamstra S. (2011) Technology-enhanced simulation for health professions education: A systematic review and meta-analysis. *JAMA* **306**(9): 978–988.

Cooper JB, Taqueti VR. (2004) A brief history of the development of mannequin simulators for clinical education and training. *Qual Saf Health Care* **13**: 11–18.

Dunn W, Murphy JG. (2008) Simulation about safety, not fantasy. *Chest* **133**(1): 6–9.

Good ML. (2003) Patient simulation for training basic and advanced clinical skills. *Med Educ* **37**(Supp 1): 14–21.

Hendrickx K, De Winter B, Jalma WT, Avonts D, Peeraer G, Wyndaele J. (2009) Learning intimate examinations with simulated patients: The evaluation of medical students' performance. *Med Teach* **31**(4): e139–e147.

Holocomb J, Dumire RD, Crommett JW, Stamateris CE, Fagert MA, Cleveland JA, Gina R, Dorlac W, Bonar JP, Hira K, Aoki N, Mattox KL. (2002) Evaluation of trauma team performance using an advanced human patient simulator for resuscitation training. *J Trauma* **52**(6): 1078–1086.

Issenberg SB, McGaghie WC, Hart IR, Mayer JW, MD, Felner JM, Petrusa ER, Waugh RA, Brown DR, Safford RS, Gessner IH, Gordon DL, MD, Ewy GA. (1999) Simulation technology for health care professional skills training and assessment. *JAMA* **282**(9): 861–866.

Lee KH, Grantham H, Boyd R. (2008) Comparison of high- and low-fidelity mannequins for clinical performance assessment. *Emerg Med Australia* **20**(6): 508–514.

Maran NJ, Glavin RJ. (2003) Low- to high-fidelity simulation — a continuum of medical education? *Med Educ* **37**(Supp 1): 22–28.

McGaghie WC, Issenberg SB, Petrusa ER, Scalese RJ. (2006) Effect of practice on standardised learning outcomes in simulation-based medical education. *Med Educ* **40**(8): 792–797.

Motola I, Devine LA, Chung HS, Sullivan JE, Issenberg SB. (2013) Simulation in healthcare education: A best evidence practical guide. AMEE Guide No. 82. *Med Teach* **35**(10): e1511–e1530.

Sengupta A, Todd AJ, Leslie SJ, Bagnall A, Boon NA, Fox KA, Denvir MA. (2007) Peer-led medical student tutorials using the cardiac simulator "Harvey". *Med Educ* **41**(2): 218–219.

Winkel AF, Lerner V, Zabar SR, Szyld D. (2013) A simple framework for assessing technical skills in a resident Observed Structured Clinical Examination (OSCE): Vaginal laceration repair. *J Surg Educ* **70**(1): 10–14.

Ziv A, Wolpe PR, Small SD, Glick S. (2003) Simulation-based medical education: An ethical imperative. *Acad Med* **78**(8): 783–788.

10

PREPARING THE GROUNDWORK FOR CONDUCTING AN OSCE

The OSCE is a complex undertaking. The design of the OSCE is such that a minor oversight might have a cascading effect on the overall examination. A badly implemented OSCE would undermine the overall credibility of the examination. We can divide the tasks to be undertaken by the organizers of an OSCE into: Actions that need to be taken before the day of the OSCE; tasks to be completed on the day of OSCE; and tasks to be completed after the OSCE.

> At the end of this chapter, we should be able to:
>
> (i) Use a structured framework for the implementation of an OSCE.
> (ii) Determine the critical practical steps that should be undertaken during the implementation of an OSCE.
> (iii) Recognize the role of the administrators and support staff in the implementation of an OSCE.

Faculty Training

Although the OSCE has existed for about four decades, there have been many variations in the way that the OSCE has been implemented around the world. There are variations in terms of purpose, format, and content of the OSCE. As expected, variations in OSCE formats also create heterogeneity and a lack of standardization. The OSCE in a specific institute may be different from another. Besides, many examiners may not have first-hand experience of developing and implementing an OSCE (van der Vleuten *et al.*, 1989).

The OSCE provides a wonderful avenue for faculty training, not only for OSCE-specific aspects, but also for general aspects of assessment (Holmboe, 2004; Pell, Homer, & Roberts, 2008). Implementation of an OSCE provides an impetus to create a broader understanding of the role of assessment among the faculty, whether they are involved as examiners or not. Faculty briefing also creates a platform for the recruitment of case writers and examiners (Fig. 10.1).

The content of faculty training workshops depends on the prior level of knowledge among the faculty and the purpose of the OSCE (de Villiers & Archer, 2012; Tan & Azila, 2007). Here is a general list of content that could be included in a faculty training workshop:

  (i) Introduction to the assessment of clinical competence;
 (ii) Basic concepts in assessment, including validity, reliability, and educational impact;
(iii) Overall assessment plan of the medical school;
(iv) Master blueprint for the entire examination;
 (v) OSCE blueprint for the clinical skills assessment;
(vi) Purpose of the OSCE;
(vii) Role of case writers in an OSCE;
(viii) Role of the examiners in an OSCE.

We also find it useful and suggest showing videos of an OSCE during the orientation. It is preferable to develop a home-grown orientation video that takes into account the unique context and cultural perspectives of the institution. In the absence of such videos, you might benefit from other institutes or from searching online. For example, the National Board of Medical Examiners

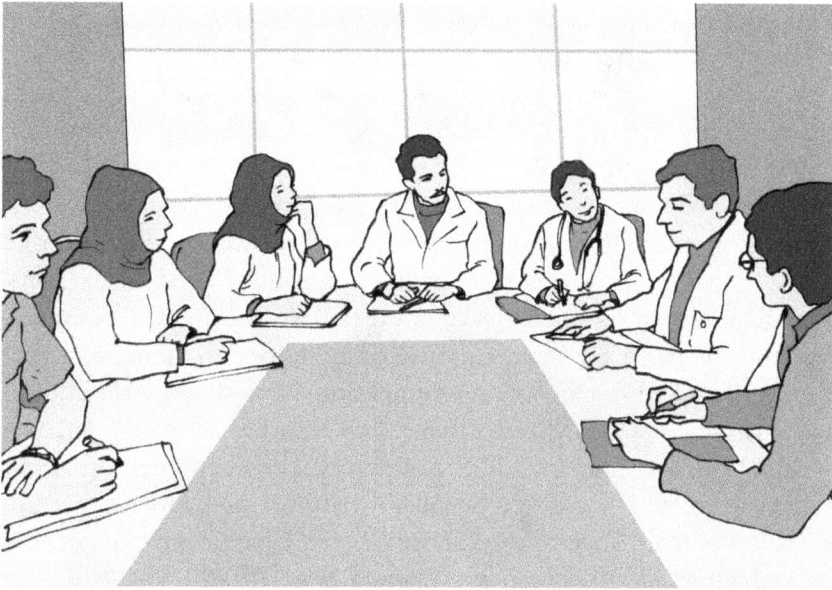

Fig. 10.1. Faculty training is necessary to prepare examiners for an OSCE.

(NBME) has a video of clinical skills assessment that might be useful as an orientation video. The video is available at http://www.usmle. org/practice-materials/index.html.

During the faculty training, encourage the faculty to work as an interdisciplinary group and develop OSCE stations. Thereafter, these OSCE stations can be used as a practice run, with the faculty taking the roles of standardized patients, students, and examiners. Such an exercise is invaluable for providing real-life experience to the faculty and to identify the many faults that are associated with OSCE station development, standardized patient training, and implementation.

Selecting Examiners for an OSCE

Selecting examiners for an OSCE can be a potentially contentious issue and is subject to much on-going discussion within the medical education community (Humprey-Murto, Touchie, & Smee, 2013). The range of potential examiners include trained lay persons, standardized patients, simulated patients, nursing and para-clinical staff, general practitioners, and specialist doctors. Some OSCE stations may not need the physical presence of examiners in the room.

The main factors that should determine the choice of examiners are: Commitment and preparedness to serve as examiners in the OSCE; ability to follow instructions; and suitability of the examiners to examine the given tasks. Studies have shown that examiner commitment to an examination is imperative in maintaining the objectivity and fairness of an examination (Wilkinson *et al.*, 2003). Both trained standardized patients and non-physicians are equally capable of serving as OSCE examiners, provided they are adequately trained and there are clear instructions on the expected level of performance by the candidates (de Champlain *et al.*, 1997; Tamblyn *et al.*, 1991; van der Vleuten *et al.*, 1989).

Arguments can be made that the OSCE stations that test high-degree clinical judgments and clinical decision-making and stations that test complex clinical skills requiring significant medical knowledge are better examined by clinicians with expert knowledge in that field. Conversely, the OSCE stations that test standardized tasks, procedural skills, and stations that can be observed and marked adequately with checklists can be examined by non-clinicians.

Use expert clinicians for the OSCE stations that:

- Test clinical judgments and medical decision-making
- Involve complex patient scenarios
- Require a high degree of medical knowledge

Consider using non-clinicians for OSCE stations that:

- Test procedural skills and simplified clinical tasks
- Test generic skills such as communication and counseling
- Can be scored with checklists

As finding an adequate number of suitable examiners in a given day is always challenging, our recommendation is to broaden the examiner pool and to always explore whether a particular station can be examined by trained lay persons or para-clinical staff rather than busy physicians. In addition, it is more meaningful to have a single examiner per station, as opposed to two examiners per station, and increase the number of stations. This approach has a better effect on the overall reliability of the OSCE (Swanson & Norcini, 1989).

Examiners' Briefing

"Even senior examiners must be prepared to dispense with personal preferences in the interests of objectivity and reproducibility and must assess students according to the marking scheme rather than rely on intuition."

Selby *et al.*, (1995)

The purposes of the examiners' briefing are to:

 (i) Orient all examiners to the upcoming OSCE;
 (ii) Provide station-specific instructions to the examiners involved;
(iii) Review station materials, including instructions to the candidate and the marking template;
(iv) Practice "live" with standardized patients (SPs);
 (v) Provide feedback to the SPs on their performance;
(vi) Agree on the minimal level of competence expected to pass the station;
(vii) Suggest specific modifications that might be necessary in the station.

It is recommended that the Module or Phase Leader or OSCE Coordinator conduct the briefing to all examiners. This is followed by a station-specific briefing by station developers or case writers to all the examiners involved in that given station. All SPs should be present during the briefing in order to demonstrate their portrayal of the case and to make necessary changes. Attendance at the examiners' briefing is mandatory for all examiners involved in the OSCE. Examiners' briefings should take place 3–7 days before the actual date of the examination in order to make any necessary modifications to the OSCE stations. If non-clinicians or non-experts are used as examiners, they may need longer briefing time than the clinician examiners, especially in stations with significant medical contents (van der Vleuten *et al.*, 1989).

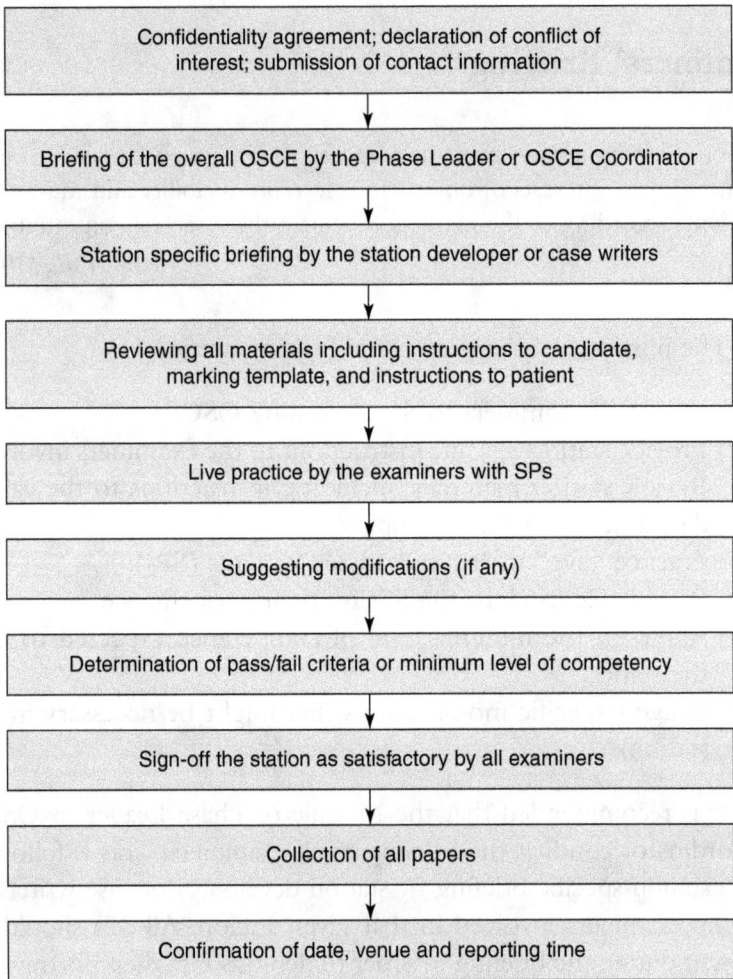

Confidentiality agreement; declaration of conflict of interest; submission of contact information

↓

Briefing of the overall OSCE by the Phase Leader or OSCE Coordinator

↓

Station specific briefing by the station developer or case writers

↓

Reviewing all materials including instructions to candidate, marking template, and instructions to patient

↓

Live practice by the examiners with SPs

↓

Suggesting modifications (if any)

↓

Determination of pass/fail criteria or minimum level of competency

↓

Sign-off the station as satisfactory by all examiners

↓

Collection of all papers

↓

Confirmation of date, venue and reporting time

Suggested flowchart of an examiners' briefing.

Students' Briefing

The students' briefing, like the examiners' briefing, is also critical for the success of the OSCE. The purposes of students' briefings are to:

(i) Orient the students to the OSCE;
(ii) Provide information on:

    (i) Examples of skills to be tested;
    (ii) The marking criteria;
    (iii) The format of the OSCE, including the:

        (i) Number of the stations;
        (ii) Station duration;
        (iii) Nature of the station;
        (iv) Rest station (if any);

    (iv) Date, time, venue of reporting;
    (v) Things to bring by the students;

(iii) Clarify students' roles and responsibilities during the OSCE.

As with the faculty briefing, preparation of an orientation video on the OSCE is highly recommended. Students may have preconceived ideas about the OSCE from prior runs or from colleagues. It is important to clarify their doubts, alleviate their fear, and project the OSCE as a more objective, more rigorous and certainly fairer examination.

Pilot Run

One of the most important elements of the successful implementation of the OSCE is pilot testing (Davis, 2003). Pilot implementation is imperative if the OSCE is to be used in high-stakes summative examinations. Pilot runs should be as realistic as possible, with the collection of structured feedback from students, examiners, and administrators.

A case study of OSCE implementation

A given medical school decided to implement the OSCE as a part of summative assessment. The school's leadership formed a taskforce for the implementation of the OSCE. The members of the taskforce attended several workshops on the OSCE. In turn, the taskforce conducted workshops for the native faculty and administrators.

Later, an experimental OSCE was conducted with a small number of invited students and faculty in order to determine its feasibility and educational value. The data from the experimental OSCE run were encouraging. This led to a full-scale pilot run with all students. Although the students were given options to opt out and they were told that the OSCE marks will not contribute towards their grade, virtually all students attended the full-scale pilot run. Pilot runs allowed the taskforce to:

- Train faculty to develop the OSCE stations;
- Create a baseline competency level among the students;
- Orient all stakeholders to the OSCE;
- Identify and expand the pool of SPs;
- Identify venues suitable for the OSCE.

Next year, the OSCE was conducted as an adjunct examination; i.e. although the marks counted towards the students' overall grades, failure in the OSCE did not jeopardize the students' overall pass grade. In other words, this OSCE was a moderately high-stakes examination. A detailed post-examination review was completed to:

- Determine the impact of the OSCE on students' overall grades;
- Triangulate marks from the OSCE with the other forms of clinical examination;
- Select the preferred method of standard setting.

A full-scale summative OSCE, replacing the traditional long cases, took place in the following year. The timeline from formation of task force to the full-scale implementation was 4 years.

Checklist for the Day of the OSCE

A checklist is a convenient way to prevent errors in the system. A checklist does not need to have all of the steps for conducting an OSCE, but it should contain all of the *critical* steps that can frequently go wrong or the steps that can have a major impact on the examination. You must develop your own checklist for the examination. An example is presented in Table 10.1.

Table 10.1.   An Example of a Checklist for the Day of the OSCE

Action	Responsibility	Done
Send SMS to all the examiners the evening before the examination		
Invite spare examiners		
Prepare spare SPs		
Rooms are equipped according to the station-specific requirements		
Rooms do not contain any unwanted materials and computer connection		
Inform examiners, candidates, and SPs to switch off mobile phones		
Bell is audible from all rooms		
Spare power sources and batteries are available		
All candidates' matriculation numbers are printed on the marking sheets		
By the end of the examination, all marking sheets are completed (no empty items) by the examiners		
All marking sheets contain the signatures of the examiners		
All marking sheets are collected		
All unnecessary examination-related materials are shredded		

OSCE Administration

In a summative examination, the accuracy of data collection and management is of paramount importance. Frequent errors in this respect include: Missing data fields in the OSCE marking sheets; misidentification of students; and incorrect data entry. If an Excel file is created for data entry, particular attention must be given to ensure that a row that is assigned to a particular student captures that specific student's mark. If the student's mark is entered into a wrong row, it is possible that all subsequent students' marks will also end up in wrong rows. Institutes may develop online examination management software to minimize the administrative burden and inherent transcriptional errors that might be associated with transferring data from a paper-and-pencil format to an electronic database. One such OSCE management software is OSCE Manager (http://www.osce-manager.com), developed by the medical faculty of the University of Basel (Switzerland). If data are manually transcribed, it is sound practice to carry out an accepted data cleaning protocol on the data that have been entered, including double entry of data or checking a random sample of data (or every n^{th} entry), until no errors are found.

Security

Needless to say, the security of examination materials in a high-stakes examination is of paramount importance. The OSCE poses a special challenge because of the many different kinds of people involved in the development of the OSCE, including administrators, lay persons, SPs, technicians, examiners, and question writers. In addition, in medical schools with a large number of candidates, it might be necessary to have several parallel sessions or several runs of OSCE circuits. In such situations, students need to be quarantined appropriately.

Recommended practice for a high-stake OSCE

- Student identification data should be preprinted on the marking sheet
- Identification data should be displayed prominently on every student
- If manual marking is used, all data should be transcribed twice (double data entry)
- All data entry should be done on an ongoing basis and completed within the day of the OSCE
- The institute may develop or implement examination management software and enter data "live" during the OSCE

Summary

High-stakes OSCE administration is a highly sophisticated exercise with considerable logistical challenges. Successful implementation of an OSCE requires meticulous forward planning, pilot testing, clear delineation of the roles and responsibilities of the different personnel involved in the OSCE, and a carefully developed checklist. Examiner training and briefing is critical for improving the validity and reliability of the examination.

References

Adamo G. (2003) Simulated and standardized patients in OSCEs: Achievements and challenges 1992–2003. *Med Teach* **25**(3): 262–270.

Boursicot K, Roberts T. (2005) How to set up an OSCE. *Clin Teach* **2**(1): 16–19.

Davis MH. (2003) OSCE: The Dundee experience. *Med Teach* **25**(3): 255–261.

de Champlain AF, Margolis MJ, King A, Klass DJ. (1997) Standardized patients' accuracy in recording examinees' behaviors using checklists. *Acad Med* **72**(10 Suppl 1): S85–S87.

de Villiers A, Archer E. (2012). The development, implementation and evaluation of a short course in objective structured clinical examination (OSCE) skills. *South African Family Practice* **54**(1): 50–54.

Hodges B. (2002) Creating, monitoring, and improving a Psychiatry OSCE: A guide for faculty. *Acad Psychiatry* **26**(3): 134–161.

Holmboe E. (2004). Faculty and observation of trainees' clinical skills: Problems and opportunities. *Acad Med* **79**(1): 16–22.

Holmboe ES, Yepes M, Williams F, Hout SJ. (2004) Feedback and mini-clinical evaluation exercise. *J Gen Intern Med* **19**(5 pt 2): 558–561.

Humprey-Murto S, Touchie C, Smee S. (2013) Objective structured clinical examination. In: Walsh K (ed.), *Oxford Textbook of Medical Education*, Oxford University Press, UK, pp. 524–536.

Pell G, Homer M, Roberts TE. (2008) Assessor training: Its effects on criterion-based assessment in a medical context. *Int J Res Method Educ* **31**(2): 143–154.

Selby C, Osman L, Davis M, Lee M. (1995) Set up and run an objective structured clinical exam. *Br Med J* **310**(6988): 1187–1190.

Swanson D, Norcini JJ. (1989) Factors influencing the reproducibility of test using standardized patients. *Teach Learn Med* **1**: 158–166.

Tamblyn RM, Klass DJ, Schnabl GK, Kopelow ML. (1991) The accuracy of standardized patient presentation. *Med Educ* **25**(2): 100–109.

Tan CP, Azila NM. (2007) Improving OSCE examiner skills in a Malaysian setting. *Med Educ* **41**(5): 517.

van der Vleuten CPM, Swanson DB. (1990) Assessment of clinical skills with standardized patients: state of the art. *Teach Learn Med* **2**(2): 58–76.

van der Vleuten CPM, van Luyk SJ, van Ballegooijen AMJ, Swansons DB. (1989) Training and experience of examiners. *Med Educ* **23**(3): 290–296.

Wilkinson TJ, Frampton CM, Thompson-Fawcett M, Egan T. (2003) Objectivity in objective structured clinical examinations: Checklists are no substitute for examiner commitment. *Acad Med* **78**(2): 219–223.

11

DETERMINING PASSES AND FAILS IN AN OSCE

This chapter details how to set the pass mark for an OSCE using the most appropriate and most commonly used method of standard setting for an OSCE.

At the end of the chapter, we should be able to:

(i) Explain the basic concepts and principles of standard setting.
(ii) Justify why the borderline group method and its variants are the most appropriate standard setting methods for an OSCE.
(iii) Apply the borderline group method for an OSCE in your own setting and arrive at an appropriate standard for an OSCE.
(iv) Critically analyze the literature on the borderline regression method of standard setting for an OSCE.

Basic Concepts and Principles of Standard Setting

Standard setting refers to determining the pass mark of an examination (Kaufman *et al.*, 2001; Norcini, 2003). This is a crucial activity in any assessment process, as this process distinguishes the candidates who are competent from those who are incompetent. Let us consider a hypothetical example. In a given OSCE station, the total mark is 20; i.e. this is the maximum mark that a candidate can obtain for this station. For this exercise, assume that the pass

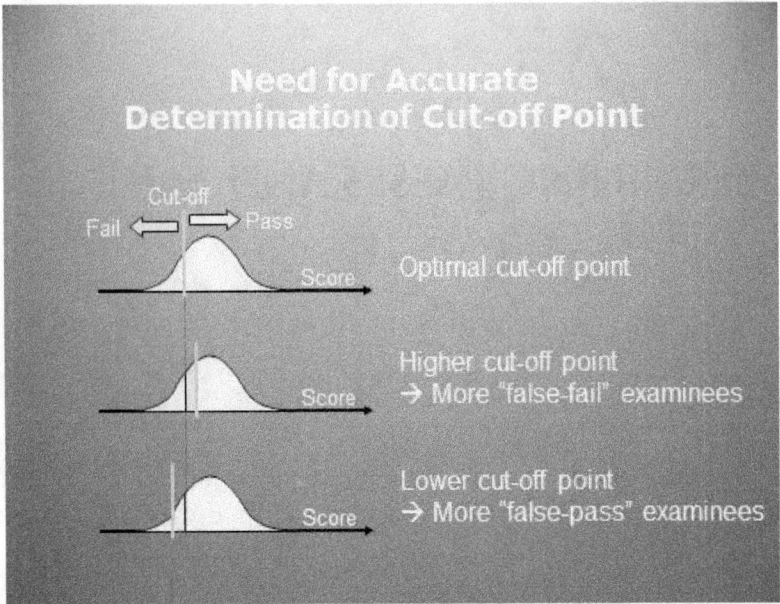

Fig. 11.1. The pass/fail distinction depends on the determination of the cut-off point. (Used with permission from Dr Hirotaka Onishi, Tokyo, Japan.)

mark for the station is set at 10, or 50% of the total. This would give rise to the following scenarios. A higher cut-off point than what would have been reasonable for the given station would result in "false-fail" candidates (Fig. 11.1). Conversely, a lower cut-off point than what would have been reasonable for the given station would result in "false-pass" candidates. The exercise of standard setting aims to minimize the number of false-pass and false-fail candidates by arriving at the most reasonable estimate of the cut-off point for a given station.

There are many strategies used to set the standard (i.e. the pass mark). They are broadly divided into four major categories.

(i) Arbitrary or fixed standards: This category of methods decides the pass mark without explicitly considering the candidate's ability or the difficulty of the assessment items (i.e. the questions or stations). Since the standard is fixed from examination to examination, the pass mark does not vary depending on the difficulty of the assessment items. Usually, the pass mark has been pre-identified and the examiners have to set questions so that an average candidate could answer correctly to achieve the said fixed pass mark. Therefore, the examiners have limited liberty to include difficult or easy questions or stations in the examination and vary the pass mark accordingly. This means that with a fixed pass mark, the overall level of difficulty of all the assessment items (i.e. the stations or questions) needs to be balanced. This is not an easy task, and hence there are reports that examination boards have had to moderate or adjust the results after finding out during the post-examination review that an unreasonable number of candidates had either passed or failed a given assessment or an assessment component. Hence, this method is not recommended as it cannot be educationally defended.

(ii) Norm-referenced standard setting: This category of methods determines the competent candidates by identifying a certain proportion (e.g. percentage) of candidates who score more than the others in a given examination (e.g. 75% of the highest-scoring candidates). The inherent disadvantage of this method is that the pass mark is determined by the ability or performance of a given cohort of candidates. As a consequence, a candidate who passes the examination with a not very able cohort of candidates may fail the same examination with a more able cohort of candidates. Hence, a pass or fail decision made through this method is not based on the ability of the candidate, but rather is based on the relative ability of the other candidates. Therefore, this method is not recommended for assessments that are used to determine competence. Rather, its use should be confined either to selection examinations, where the intake has to be limited to the number of training slots available, or to instances where the awarding of medals and prizes to the best candidates is necessary.

(iii) Criterion-referenced standard setting: This category of standard setting determines the pass mark by relating the materials that are being assessed to the ability of a candidate who is at the threshold of passing or failing. Such a candidate is called the "borderline candidate." Technically, the "borderline candidate" is defined as the candidate who has a 50% probability (or chance) of passing or failing. Thus, the pass mark set by the methods within this category of standard setting is directly related to the expected ability level of the candidate. Since the standard that is set by these methods of standard setting is not dependent on the ability of the cohort of candidates, these methods overcome the main disadvantage (i.e. the pass mark varying from one cohort of candidates to another) of norm-referenced standard setting. As such, these methods are also called "absolute" standard setting methods. Hence, for competency-based assessment, this is the preferred method of standard setting.

Criterion-referenced methods have two basic approaches based on the focus upon which the standard setting process concentrates.

(i) Test-centered methods: This group of methods focuses on the difficulty of each assessment item (usually in relation to the borderline candidate) in order to determine the pass mark. Examples include the Angoff method, the modified Angoff method, the Ebel method, the Jaegre method, etc. The advantage of this group of methods is that the pass mark can be set before the examination is held. The main disadvantage is that since the standard setters have to work hypothetically, rather than based on actual examination results, the pass mark is susceptible to becoming unrealistic, at least in certain instances.

(ii) Examinee-centered methods: These methods focus on the ability (i.e. the scores) of the candidates when determining the pass mark. Examples include the borderline group method and the contrasting groups method. The main advantage of this group of methods is that examiners work with the actual candidates in order to determine the pass mark. Therefore, there is a lesser chance of the pass mark becoming unrealistic. In addition, the examiners (i.e. the standard setters) need to spend less time prior to the examination in order to determine the pass mark. The main disadvantage, however, is that the pass mark will only be known after the examination.

(iv) Compromise methods: This type of method attempts to combine the advantages of both the norm- and criterion-referenced methods, while trying to mitigate their individual disadvantages (e.g. the Hofstee method).

Of these four methods, the borderline group method, which is an examinee-centered method, is the preferred method for standard setting in an OSCE.

Classical Borderline Group Method of Standard Setting

To set the pass mark using the classical borderline group method, each OSCE station has to be marked using a checklist and a global rating scale (see Chapter 7). The global rating scale is used to identify the borderline candidates. The average (or median) checklist mark for all of the borderline candidates (as identified by the global rating scale) is then calculated and considered as the pass mark for the said station.

Hence, the steps for carrying out the borderline group method of standard setting can be explained as below (Fig. 11.2).

If the examination board wants the candidates to pass each and every station, then each station can set a pass mark as in Step 3; i.e. Step 4 is not necessary. However, if the examination board only wants the candidates to achieve a single pass mark for the entire OSCE (i.e. for all of the stations), then Step 4 should be carried out. The former (i.e. stipulating that the candidates need to achieve the

Step 1: **Before the** **OSCE**	**Examiners' meeting:** The examiners meet and discuss in order to arrive at a consensus as to the characteristics of a borderline candidate. They lead the discussion based on their experience in teaching, supervising, and examining candidates at the level of ability that the OSCE purports to assess. Hence, it goes without saying that all examiners (i.e. standard setters) need to be experienced clinicians or teachers who have taught, supervised, and assessed candidates of a similar ability level.
Step 2: **During the** **OSCE**	**Scoring candidate ability:** The examiners mark each candidate using both the checklist and the global rating scale. It is important that the examiners consider the checklist and the global rating scale separately and use the two marking instruments (i.e. the checklist and the global rating scale) independently.
Step 3: **After the OSCE**	**Pass mark per station:** The checklist marks of all of the candidates of a given station that the examiners mark as 'borderline' on the global rating scale are averaged in order to arrive at the pass mark for the station.
Step 4 **Deciding the** **standard**	**Pass mark for the OSCE:** The pass marks for all of the stations, which are established by following steps 1 to 3, are then summed up (and averaged if necessary) in order to arrive at the pass mark for the entire OSCE. Some examination boards add one standard error of measurement to this pass mark in order to minimize the false positives.

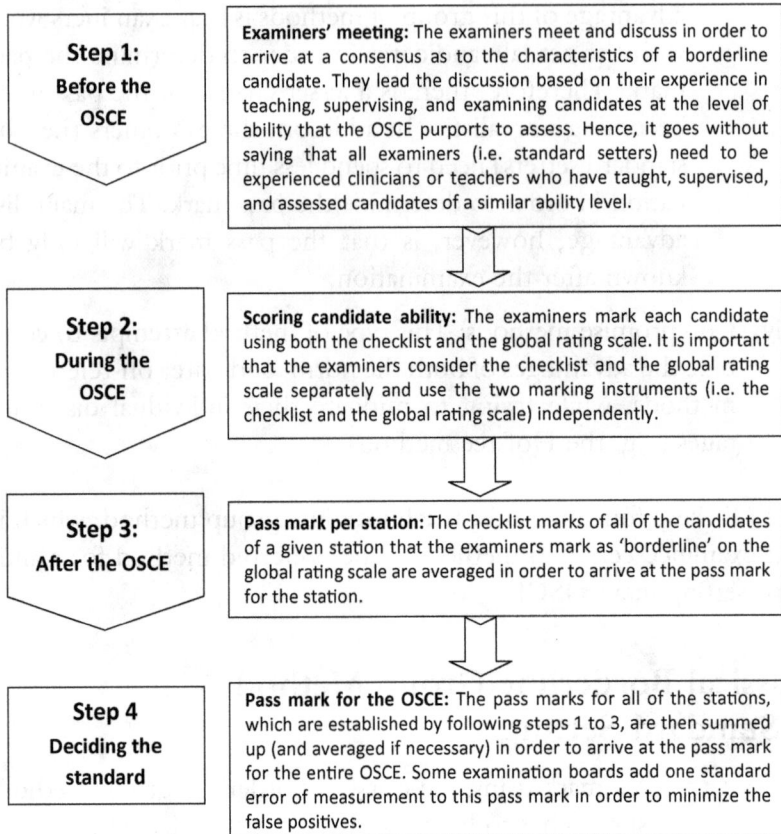

Fig. 11.2.   The process of classical borderline group standard setting for an OSCE.

individual pass mark for each and every station) is called "conjunctive standards," while the latter (i.e. allowing the candidates to mitigate a poor score at one station with an excellent score at another station) is called "compensatory standards." Since conjunctive standards lead to higher failure rates, the usual practice is to use conjunctive standards sparingly (i.e. only when it is absolutely essential).

> The usual practice is to set compensatory standards. However, conjunctive standards could be applied to certain stations that assess life-saving skills, such as a station on cardiopulmonary resuscitation.

Below is a set of marks from an OSCE station. Twenty candidates were assessed at this station, and each candidate was scored using a checklist and a global rating scale. The global rating scale is a five-point Likert scale, where 3 is identified as the "borderline" rating point. The checklist has 10 items of 1 mark each.

Candidate no.	Checklist Total	Global
1	4	3
2	5	3
3	2	2
4	6	3
5	7	4
6	1	1
7	9	5
8	6	4
9	6	3
10	4	3
11	7	4
12	8	4
13	3	2
14	3	1
15	2	2
16	7	4
17	5	3
18	1	1
19	10	5
20	2	3

The global rating scale is as follows:

1	2	3	4	5
Very poor	Poor	Borderline	Good	Excellent

Can You Calculate the Pass Mark for this Station?

Answer: In this example, candidates 1, 2, 4, 9, 10, 17, and 20 have been identified by the examiners as borderline candidates through the global rating scale. The average checklist mark for these candidates can thus be calculated as follows:

Average checklist mark for borderline candidates = (4 + 5 + 6 + 6 + 4 + 5 + 2)/7 = 32/7 = 4.57 out of 10

Therefore, 5 out of 10 marks can be considered to be the pass mark for this station.

Limitations of the Classical Borderline Group Method

(i) To arrive at a defensible pass mark, this method requires an adequate number of candidates and an adequate number of examiners (Pell *et al.*, 2010; Pell & Roberts, 2006). Hence, this method was traditionally used for large multicenter OSCEs, which had around 1000 candidates and, due to multiple OSCE circuits, multiple examiners for the same station. However, more recently, this method has also been used in examinations that have a lesser number of candidates (e.g. around 200 candidates).

(ii) Even with a reasonable number of candidates, there may be the possibility (at least hypothetically) that a given station may not have any borderline candidate at the end of the entire OSCE. In this case, the pass mark could not be worked out by this method for such a station.

Therefore, in order to overcome these disadvantages, the borderline regression method, which uses the scores of all of the candidates, not just the borderline candidates, is preferred.

Borderline Regression Method

The conduct of the standard setting process as outlined in Steps 1 and 2 in Fig. 11.2 is the same for this method as well. Only the calculation of the pass mark is different.

Here, the scores of all of the candidates are entered into a simple linear regression model, where the independent variable is the "global rating" and the dependent variable is the "checklist total". Then, using the regression plot or using the regression equation, it is possible to calculate the checklist total (y-axis) when the global rating (x-axis) is 3; i.e. the borderline rating.

Figure 11.3 illustrates a determination using the borderline regression method for the candidate scores of the OSCE station that was considered for the classical borderline group method earlier.

As can be seen, the pass mark is approximately 5 out of 10. The pass mark, however, can also be calculated more accurately using the regression formula for this plot.

$$y = mX + C$$

$$y = (2 \times 3) + (-1.1) = 6 - 1.1$$

$$y = 4.9$$

Therefore, the pass mark for this station is 4.9 (approximately 5, as fractional marks are not awarded for this station) out of 10.

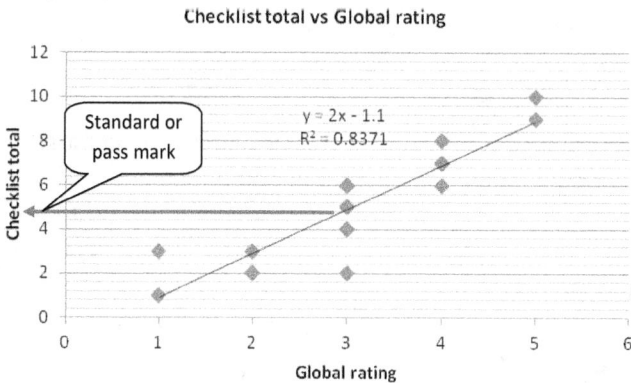

Fig. 11.3.   The regression plot for the borderline regression method.

Summary

The criterion-referenced category of standard setting is the method of choice for a competency-based, summative OSCE. The borderline group family of standard setting, which represents criterion-referenced, examinee-centered standard setting, is the most appropriate for setting the pass mark for an OSCE. The borderline group method of standard setting is simple to calculate and works well in most situations. The borderline regression method is a more statistically sophisticated method that should produce more defensible standards. Applying compensatory standards is the norm. However, conjunctive standards could be applied for certain stations, if there are compelling reasons.

References

Friedman Ben-David M. (2000) AMEE Guide No. 18: Standard setting in student assessment. *Med Teach* **22**(2): 120–130.

Kaufman DM, Mann KV, Muijtjens AMM, van der Vleuten CPM. (2000) A comparison of standard setting procedures for an OSCE in undergraduate medical education. *Acad Med* **75**(3): 267–271.

Kramer A, Muijtjens A, Jansen K, Dusman H, Tan L, van der Vleuten C. (2003) Comparison of a rational and an empirical standard setting procedure for an OSCE. *Med Educ* **37**(2): 132–137.

Norcini JJ. (2003) Setting standards on educational tests. *Med Educ* **37**(5): 464–469.

Pell G, Roberts TE. (2006) Setting standards for student assessment. *Int J Res Method Educ* **31**(2): 143–154.

Pell G, Fuller R, Homer M, Roberts T. (2010) How to measure quality of the OSCE: A review of metrics: AMEE guide no. 49. *Med Teach* **32**(10): 802–811.

Smee SM, Blackmore DE. (2001) Setting standards for an OSCE. *Med Educ* **35**(11): 1009–1010.

Wilkinson TJ, Newble DI, Frampton C. (2001) Standard setting in an objective structured clinical examination: Use of global ratings of borderline performance to determine the passing score. *Med Educ* **35**(11): 1043–1049.

12

POST-ASSESSMENT QUALITY ASSURANCE

Once an OSCE is completed, as with any assessment, it is imperative that those who were responsible for the organization and administration of the OSCE (i.e. the examination board) determine whether the OSCE has functioned as intended (Pell *et al.*, 2010, Roberts *et al.*, 2006). This could be achieved by combining various psychometric or quantitative data and non-psychometric or qualitative data. Psychometric parameters refer to the analysis of the scores of the candidates and the assessment content (Wass, McGibbon, & van der Vleuten, 2001). Item analysis is one of the most useful ways of analyzing the psychometric data of an OSCE. Commonly used qualitative data refer to candidates' feedback, examiners' feedback, and patients' feedback.

At the end of this chapter, we should be able to:

(i) Propose a framework of analysis of an OSCE, taking into consideration both psychometric and non-psychometric data.
(ii) Conduct an item analysis for an OSCE station.
(iii) Determine the nature of the qualitative data needed in order to ensure the quality of an OSCE.

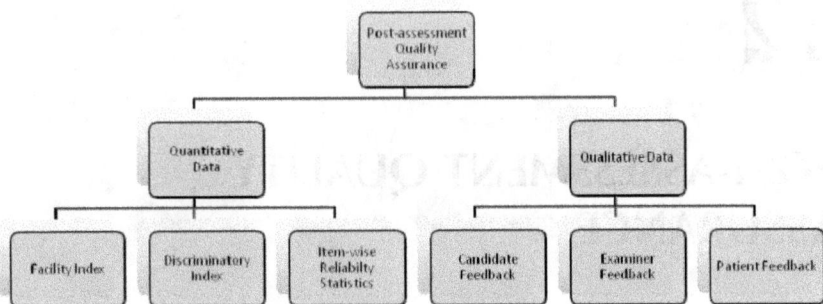

Fig. 12.1.   Post-assessment evaluation methods.

Quantitative Data (Item Analysis)

Item analysis is carried out to answer questions how good is the performance of each OSCE station. Item analysis, however, only informs how each and every assessment item (i.e. OSCE station) performed at the examination. Thus, the information obtained from item analysis should be supplemented by other evidence (e.g. feedback from the candidates and examiners, analysis of the total score, etc), which will be discussed later in this chapter, in order to provide a holistic view of the overall examination (Pell *et al.*, 2010).

It is important to differentiate the performance of an OSCE station from the performance of candidates. As the objective of item analysis is to evaluate the performance of each OSCE station, as a rule, item analysis can only be carried out after the assessment (i.e. only when the candidate scores are available). Under item analysis, we will discuss three basic psychometric parameters or indicators in relation to the OSCE that every assessment should be informed by:

(i) The facility (or difficulty) index;
(ii) The discrimination index;
(iii) Item-wise reliability statistics.

Facility Index

The facility index is traditionally called the "difficulty index." However, the name "difficulty index" is a misnomer, as a high difficulty index means that the question is easy, and vice versa. So, it is really a measure of the "easiness" of a given assessment item (i.e. the easiness of an OSCE station). Therefore, a more appropriate term is "facility index."

The facility index is calculated as the proportion of candidates who have passed (i.e. obtained scores that indicate competence) in a given OSCE station.

$$\text{Facility index} = \frac{\text{Number of candidates passing the station}}{\text{Total number of candidates sitting the OSCE}}$$

Hence, the facility index could range from 0 (absolutely difficult; nobody passed) to 1 (absolutely easy; everyone passed). If a higher proportion of candidates pass an OSCE, the facility or the easiness of the station is greater. As a rule of thumb, assessment items with a facility index of less than 0.3 are considered difficult, while a facility index of more than 0.7 represents an easy assessment item (Anonymous, 2008).

Discrimination Index

The discrimination index indicates how well an assessment item (i.e. an OSCE station) can differentiate the more able candidates from the rest. There are two methods to calculate the discrimination index. In one method, all of the candidates are ordered according to their *total* examination score. Then, for a given station, the proportion of candidates who passed this station but who are in the lower one-third of candidates according to the total examination scores is subtracted from the proportion of candidates passing the same station within the upper one-third.

$$\text{Discrimination index} = \begin{pmatrix} \text{Proportion of} \\ \text{candidates in the} \\ \text{upper 1/3 passing} \\ \text{the OSCE station} \end{pmatrix} - \begin{pmatrix} \text{Proportion of} \\ \text{candidates in the} \\ \text{lower 1/3 passing} \\ \text{the OSCE station} \end{pmatrix}$$

In the other method of calculating the discrimination index, the candidate score for a given station is correlated with the total score (of all stations, except the station under consideration) of that candidate using the standard Pearson's correlation. Hence, this method is also called item-total correlation or the point-biserial.

Discrimination index = | Pearson's correlation coefficient between the station score and the total score, without the station under investigation

Whichever the method, the logic behind this index is that a candidate who does well at the entire assessment should also do well at any given station, and vice versa. Thus, a higher value of this index indicates a higher ability of that station to separate the more able candidates from the rest.

However, of the two methods, the latter method is considered to be a superior measure, as it takes into account the scores of all the candidates, while the former only considers the scores of candidates who are in the upper and lower thirds in their rank order. This being said, when using the former method, it is easier to interpret the index.

The scale of the index (irrespective of the method) ranges from -1 (very poor discrimination) to $+1$ (excellent discrimination). Zero indicates that similar proportions of candidates are passing in both the lower and upper one-thirds, or there is no correlation between the candidate's station score and the total score of all stations (except the station under consideration) for the same candidate. This, therefore, indicates poor discrimination, but could be justified if all of the candidates have passed a station that assesses a basic, essential competence that all candidates (good or bad) should have mastered (e.g. a cardiopulmonary resuscitation station). However, a negative discrimination index is unacceptable, as it implies that the lower-ranked participants (as judged by the entire examination) have performed better than the higher-ranked participants. If so, it is likely that there may be an item construction flaw.

The cut-off values for discrimination index analyses are: >0.35 (high); 0.2–0.35 (moderate); and <0.2 (poor) (Hingorjo & Jaleel, 2012).

Item-wise Reliability Statistics

The item-wise reliability statistics are a measure that estimates how much an item (i.e. OSCE station) has contributed to the overall reliability of the examination. It is calculated by removing each item (i.e. station) one at a time, and recalculating the reliability coefficient. Since this is essentially a reliability estimate, the scale would range from 0 to 1. This can be calculated using the "alpha-if-item-deleted" function of SPSS (Statistical Package for Social Sciences). "Alpha" in this function refers to Cronbach's alpha coefficient.

So, to interpret the item-wise reliability statistics, one has to compare the item-wise reliability estimate with the overall reliability (calculated without removing the score of any station). If the alpha-if-item-deleted estimate is greater than the overall reliability coefficient, then the removed station has pulled down the overall reliability of the examination. This means that the said station lowers the overall reliability of the OSCE. That is, in the context of the entire OSCE, this station can be considered to be low in reliability.

Interpreting the Three Indicators in Unison

The decision as to whether an item has less than the expected desirability should be taken by interpreting the value of a given indicator using the methods and the criteria given under each indicator described above. However, the decision as to whether an item (i.e. station) should be reviewed before item banking should be taken only after considering all three indicators.

The only exception to this rule is when the discrimination index is negative. In such a situation, even if the other two indicators (i.e. facility index and item-wise reliability statistic) are acceptable, the item should be reviewed. In any other situation, the items that all three indicators flag up as undesirable should be considered for reviewing first. The items that two indicators flag up as undesirable should next be considered for reviewing. An item that is flagged up by only one indicator (other than a negative discrimination index) as unacceptable should be considered for revision only if there is a compelling reason. This is because the three indicators complement each other, as they share the same psychometric basis or rationale. For example, a station with an unacceptably high or low facility index is likely to have a low discrimination index. In the case of a station with a low facility index, all/most candidates (both high and low rankers) may fail the station due to the high level of difficulty. In the case of a station with a high facility index, all/most candidates may pass the station due to the high level of easiness of the station. Similarly, a station that decreases the overall reliability of the examination will have item construction flaws that would make it impossible for either the low and higher achievers to interpret the station uniformly. This again will result in a low (or even a negative) discrimination index, while the facility index may also be lower than expected. So, one undesirable index value usually means that many indices are likely to be affected.

Table 12.1 is a true set of data. We should now be able to calculate the three parameters discussed in this chapter. Consider the pass mark of each OSCE station to be 5 out of 10. Can you decide which items should be reconsidered? Please find the answers immediately below the data set. You will have to rotate the page 90° to read the answers.

In the example above, Station 11, due to its negative discrimination index (in addition to the poor alpha-if-item-deleted statistic), must be reviewed and modified or discarded.

Station 6 and Station 15 may be reconsidered for review, as all three indices are relatively poor. Due to the relative difficulty of these two stations (i.e. their low facility index), it would have been logical to expect a higher discrimination index, meaning that only the good candidates would score highly at these station. However, this is not the case. Therefore, it is more likely that these two stations may have an item construction flaw(s). This is also reflected by the alpha-if-item-deleted statistic of these two stations.

Table 12.1.   A True Set of OSCE Data

No.	St.1	St.2	St.3	St.4	St.5	St.6	St.7	St.8	St.9	St.10	St.11	St.12	St.13	St.14	St.15	St.16	St.17	St.18	St.19	St.20
1	10	10	10	10	10	10	5	10	10	10	3	3	5	10	0	5	10	10	10	10
2	10	10	10	10	10	10	5	5	6	5	10	6	10	10	0	5	10	10	5	10
3	6	10	10	10	10	10	5	5	10	10	10	10	5	10	0	10	10	10	0	0
4	10	10	6	6	10	0	5	10	10	10	6	10	10	10	0	5	0	6	10	10
5	6	10	6	10	10	10	5	10	10	10	10	6	5	10	0	5	10	6	5	0
6	6	10	6	6	10	10	0	10	5	10	10	6	5	0	10	5	10	3	10	10
7	10	6	10	3	10	10	0	10	10	10	10	6	5	10	0	10	0	6	10	0
8	6	10	6	3	10	0	5	5	5	5	6	6	10	10	0	10	10	10	5	10
9	10	10	6	3	6	0	0	10	5	10	3	6	10	10	10	5	10	6	5	10
10	6	10	10	10	10	0	10	5	10	5	6	3	5	10	10	10	0	6	5	10
11	10	10	6	6	10	0	5	5	6	10	3	6	5	10	0	10	5	10	10	0
12	10	10	0	0	10	10	10	5	5	10	10	10	5	10	0	0	10	10	0	0
13	6	3	10	3	10	0	5	0	5	5	6	6	10	0	10	5	10	6	5	0
14	6	6	6	6	10	10	5	10	10	10	10	10	0	0	10	5	10	6	5	0
15	10	10	10	3	10	0	0	0	5	10	6	6	10	10	0	10	0	6	5	0
16	10	10	3	3	0	0	10	5	0	10	10	10	5	10	0	10	10	10	5	0
17	10	10	10	6	0	0	5	0	10	10	6	5	5	0	10	10	10	10	5	0
18	10	6	6	6	0	0	10	5	5	5	3	6	10	0	10	10	10	10	0	0
19	6	10	10	10	0	0	0	0	10	10	6	3	10	10	5	5	0	10	5	0

(Continued)

Table 12.1.   (*Continued*)

No.	St.1	St.2	St.3	St.4	St.5	St.6	St.7	St.8	St. 9	St.10	St.11	St.12	St.13	St.14	St.15	St.16	St.17	St.18	St.19	St.20
20	6	10	3	3	10	0	10	10	10	5	6	6	10	10	0	10	10	0	0	0
21	10	10	6	6	10	0	5	0	10	10	6	10	10	0	10	10	6	0	0	0
22	10	10	6	10	6	0	0	0	10	10	10	6	10	10	0	0	10	5	0	0
23	6	10	10	6	10	0	5	5	10	5	10	3	10	10	0	10	3	5	0	0
24	6	10	3	6	10	0	0	10	10	5	10	5	5	10	0	10	10	5	0	0
25	6	10	6	3	10	10	0	0	10	5	6	3	5	10	10	0	6	5	10	10
26	10	10	6	0	6	10	0	10	5	5	6	10	10	0	0	10	10	5	0	0
27	6	10	6	3	10	0	5	5	3	5	6	3	5	10	10	10	10	5	0	0
28	10	10	3	3	10	0	5	10	10	10	3	3	10	10	0	0	3	10	10	0
29	10	10	6	3	10	0	0	10	10	5	10	6	5	10	10	10	10	5	0	0
30	10	10	6	3	10	0	0	0	10	10	10	10	0	0	10	10	10	0	0	0
31	10	6	10	6	10	0	5	10	5	5	10	6	5	0	10	0	6	5	0	0
32	10	10	10	6	10	0	0	10	5	10	6	6	10	0	0	0	10	5	0	0
33	10	10	3	3	10	10	5	0	10	10	6	6	5	0	0	0	10	10	0	0
34	6	10	3	6	6	0	5	5	10	5	6	6	0	10	0	10	10	10	5	0
35	10	10	3	6	6	0	0	5	10	5	6	6	5	0	0	10	10	5	0	10
36	3	10	10	6	3	0	0	0	10	10	3	10	0	0	10	5	10	10	10	0
37	10	6	10	6	10	10	5	0	5	5	6	6	5	0	10	0	6	0	0	0

(*Continued*)

Table 12.1. (Continued)

No.	St.1	St.2	St.3	St.4	St.5	St.6	St.7	St.8	St.9	St.10	St.11	St.12	St.13	St.14	St.15	St.16	St.17	St.18	St.19	St.20
38	10	10	3	3	6	0	0	0	10	10	10	10	0	10	0	5	0	10	10	0
39	6	10	3	3	10	0	6	0	5	10	6	3	5	10	0	5	10	10	5	0
40	3	6	6	10	10	0	5	0	5	10	10	10	0	0	0	10	0	10	0	10
41	6	0	6	6	10	10	0	0	5	5	10	3	5	0	0	5	10	10	10	0
42	6	6	10	6	6	0	5	0	10	10	10	3	10	10	0	0	0	3	0	10
43	10	10	0	0	10	10	5	0	5	10	6	3	0	0	0	5	10	6	10	0
44	10	6	10	3	6	0	5	5	10	10	6	3	5	10	0	5	0	6	5	0
45	6	0	3	0	6	0	0	0	10	10	6	10	10	0	0	10	0	10	5	0
46	10	10	3	0	10	10	0	0	0	5	6	10	5	10	0	5	10	10	0	0
47	6	0	10	6	10	0	10	0	0	5	6	6	5	10	0	0	10	6	0	0
48	10	10	0	3	10	10	0	5	5	10	6	0	0	10	0	5	0	10	0	0
49	10	6	6	6	10	0	0	0	5	5	3	3	10	0	0	5	0	10	0	0
50	6	10	6	0	0	0	0	10	10	5	10	6	10	0	5	0	0	3	0	0
51	6	10	6	10	10	0	0	5	5	5	6	3	0	0	0	5	0	10	0	0
52	6	6	0	0	3	0	0	0	5	5	6	6	10	0	0	5	0	3	0	0

Station	St.1	St.2	St.3	St.4	St.5	St.6	St.7	St.8	St.9	St.10	St.11	St.12	St.13	St.14	St.15	St.16	St.17	St.18	St.19	St.20
Discrimination	0.08	0.15	0.38	0.23	0.15	0.23	0.46	0.62	0.15	0.00	−0.15	0.38	0.31	0.54	0.23	0.15	0.38	0.15	0.46	0.38
Facility	0.96	0.92	0.75	0.56	0.92	0.31	0.54	0.58	0.90	1.00	0.87	0.71	0.83	0.60	0.33	0.92	0.58	0.88	0.67	0.21
Alpha-if-item-deleted (alpha = 0.40)	0.40	0.37	0.34	0.35	0.36	0.42	0.37	0.36	0.40	0.38	0.42	0.40	0.42	0.37	0.45	0.39	0.40	0.41	0.36	0.37

Shaded in darker grey is a station that *must* be reviewed and modified, while shaded in lighter grey are the stations that *could* be reviewed.

Station 18, on the other hand, has a very poor discrimination index, but this may be justified as a station testing an essential area in the curriculum that all candidates should be proficient with. This explanation would have been appropriate had the alpha-if-item-deleted statistic been favorable. However, the balance is tipped negatively due to the less than ideal alpha-if-item-deleted statistic.

Station 13, on the other hand, is an easy question (with a high facility index), but with a moderately high discrimination index. Once again, the balance may be tipped against this station due to the poor alpha-if-item-deleted statistic.

Station 10, despite its discrimination index of 0, can be interpreted as a station that tests a mandatory (or essential) area in the curriculum that all candidates should have mastered (e.g. a cardiopulmonary resuscitation station), mainly due to the 100% facility.

Item Analysis Using Advanced Psychometric Theories

It should be stressed that the results of all of the above three psychometric techniques of items analysis would be dependent upon the cohort of candidates of whom the results are being analyzed. Thus, the item statistics may differ significantly if the same test items are administered to another cohort of candidates, especially if the cohort size is small. Hence, it would be ideal to have a psychometric technique that would determine the item statistics independently of the cohort that takes the test items. Item response theory and its variants (e.g. Rasch modeling) offer such techniques. Similarly, more information about the reliability of the OSCE, such as the contributory factors to the reliability of the OSCE, and the number of stations and examiners per station that would optimize reliability could be obtained using the generalizability theory. It is beyond the scope of this manual to detail these theories. However, suffice it to say that, for the advanced practitioner, there are methods and techniques to evaluate test items more scientifically. This being said, it should be also emphasized that continuously calculating the three parameters discussed in detail in this chapter at each administration of an assessment should provide sound enough information for making the crucial decisions.

Qualitative Data (Feedback)

Quantitative data about the quality of the OSCE should be supplemented with qualitative data collected from key stakeholders. Three common sources of qualitative data for evaluating an OSCE are candidates, examiners, and patients (standardized or simulated). In addition, feedback on the overall conduct of the OSCE can be collected from the administrators.

Feedback from Candidates

Feedback from candidates is perhaps the most important feedback that we can collect regarding the quality of the OSCE. The purpose of this feedback is not to criticize each and every OSCE station. Rather, it is to collect information on how the OSCE can be improved further. The best time to collect this feedback is immediately after the OSCE is finished. Feedback can be collected on the overall OSCE or on individual stations. The key questions that the candidates should be asked, are:

(i) Did the OSCE match the learning outcomes detailed in the curriculum?

(ii) Were the tasks important for your future functioning as a doctor?

(iii) Were the skills that were tested in the OSCE taught in the curriculum?

(iv) Was the overall difficulty of the OSCE appropriate for the level of training?

(v) Were the instructions to the candidate clear?

(vi) Was the time sufficient to complete the tasks?

(vii) Did the simulated patient perform appropriately?

(viii) Do you have any specific suggestion for improving the OSCE?

Feedback from Examiners

Examiners should provide station-specific feedback on the quality of the OSCE station. This is in addition to qualitative comments that examiners are required to make on the scoring template about individual candidates. Key questions that should be asked from the examiners are:

(i) Was the task in your OSCE station important for candidates' future functioning as a doctor?
(ii) Did the standardized patient portray the task realistically?
(iii) Did the patient scenario appropriately cover the salient points of the case?
(iv) Did you notice any recurring deficiencies among the candidates?
(v) Did the candidate have sufficient time to complete the tasks?
(vi) Did the scoring template capture all of the important tasks?
(vii) Was the mark distribution among the items reasonable?
(viii) Can you suggest any other skills that could be included in the future OSCE?

Feedback from Simulated Patients

Simulated patients should also provide station-specific feedback. Key questions that should be asked from the patients are:

(i) Did you find the portrayal of the case difficult?
(ii) Did you notice any recurring deficiencies among the candidates?
(iii) Did the candidates ask questions that you could not answer?
(iv) Did you receive adequate training for the role?
(v) Did any uncomfortable incident(s) happen during the station? If so, what were they?
(vi) Are you willing to volunteer again as a simulated patient? If not, why?
(vii) Did the organizers look after your needs (e.g. food, drinks, resting time, etc) as you expected?

Utilization of Data

Crucial decisions about the quality of an OSCE station should be based on the triangulation of all data. Generally speaking, unless a glaring deficiency is evident, it is our recommendation not to make crucial decisions about the quality of an OSCE based on a single data source. The quality assurance process is not complete unless the data gathered from the process and the conclusions drawn are utilized effectively for further improvement and critical actions. In addition to improving the OSCE, the data could be used for important functions and decisions, such as:

(i)   Curriculum improvement;
(ii) Moderation of marks, if needed;
(iii) Feedback to the candidates;
(iv) Banking of OSCE stations.

In the next chapter, we shall discuss these in greater detail.

Summary

The quality assurance process for an OSCE should be designed prospectively and implemented methodically. Both quantitative and qualitative data can be used to make a holistic judgment about the quality of an OSCE. Once the evaluation of the OSCE stations is completed, the suitable stations should be banked methodically for future use, and important feedback should be transmitted to the curriculum team and the examination team for further action.

References

Anonymous. (2008) A user's guide to brilliant test scoring and item analysis. Available at: http://occs.odu.edu/instruction/opscan/brilliant!_test_scoring.pdf (Accessed on 8 August 2013).

Hingorjo MR, Jaleel F. (2012) Analysis of one-best MCQs: The difficulty index, discrimination Index and distractor efficiency. *J Pak Med Assoc* **62**(2): 142–147.

Pell G, Fuller R, Homer M, Roberts T. (2010) How to measure quality of the OSCE: A review of metrics: AMEE guide no. 49. *Med Teach* **32**(10): 802–810.

Roberts C, Newble D, Jolly B. Reed M, Hampton K. (2006) Assuring the quality of high-stakes undergraduate assessment of clinical competence. *Med Teach* **28**(6): 535–543.

Wass V, McGibbon D, van der Vleuten CPM. (2001) Composite undergraduate clinical examinations: How should the components be combined to maximize reliability? *Med Educ* **35**(4): 326–330.

13

FEEDBACK, MODERATION, AND BANKING

In Chapter 12, we discussed how quantitative and qualitative data can help us in the quality assurance of an OSCE. We also learned that data from the quality assurance process can be used for various purposes. In this chapter, we expand the discussion on how the data from an OSCE can be utilized for the improvement of the curriculum, improvement of students' performance, moderation of marking (if needed), and banking of OSCE stations.

At the end of this chapter, we should be able to:

(i) Provide feedback to the curriculum committee based on quality assurance results.
(ii) Provide feedback to the candidates in order to improve their future performance.
(iii) Discuss guidelines for the moderation of marking.
(iv) Select OSCE stations that are suitable for banking.
(v) Develop a systematic process of data collection for banking.

Feedback to the Curriculum Committee

One of the crucial tasks for the OSCE team is to share the data derived during the quality assurance process with the curriculum committee. You should be able to identify a recurring pattern of deficiency of certain skills that was evident in the OSCE. The deficiency could be very specific, such as an inability to measure injectable insulin with the right syringe or failure to perform hand hygiene before and after touching the patients. Sometimes the deficiency could be more generic in nature, such as poor communication skills or poor clinical reasoning skills. It is also possible to identify a deficiency of a given rotation by studying the variability of clinical experience among the students.

Feedback to the Candidate

Feedback is one of the most important modulators of human behavior (Branch & Paranjape, 2002). Data generated during the OSCE on students' behavior, competency, and knowledge should be transmitted systematically to the students for future improvement. The focus of the feedback and debriefing session should not be criticism of student performance. Rather, the primary objective of feedback is to improve students' learning. Feedback after an OSCE is associated with better student performance (Khan *et al.*, 1997).

During the OSCE, both qualitative (written comments from the examiners) and quantitative (itemized rating scale scores) data can be collected. It is our recommendation that the OSCE marking sheet should be designed in such a way that it captures both the qualitative comments as well as quantitative data. Examiners should be encouraged to provide brief written comments, both positive and negative, on the candidates.

Feedback should be given to individual students. Individualized feedback is especially important for poorly performing students in order to develop a customized remedial plan (see Chapter 14). Group or cohort feedback is also important in order to rectify any recurring deficiencies among the students. For example, if it is noted that the students are inconsistent in hand hygiene practice during the OSCE, this should be pointed out to the students for remediation.

Although the general recommendation is to conduct student feedback and debriefing immediately after the assessment, it would be more realistic and appropriate to hold the feedback session soon after the post-examination review.

Moderation of Marks

In a carefully conducted OSCE, there should not be any need for the moderation or adjustment of marks. The accepted practice should be to review the stations thoroughly before the OSCE in order to minimize any need for moderation. However, during the review process, it is possible to identify a serious flaw with a certain station. In such situations, the Board of Examiners may recommend moderation of marks. Moderation, if needed, must take place before the marks are released to the students.

☝ Good to Know

Moderation versus scaling: Moderation is the careful and deliberate process by which the Board of Examiners adjusts the marks in order to compensate for serious faults in the examination. This is different from a large-scale arbitrary addition or deletion of marks in the examination. The latter process, unsound and unjustified, is better known as scaling or shifting.

During the quality assurance process, it might be evident that a particular station was grossly deficient or the skills tested in the OSCE were not taught in the curriculum. In such a situation, there is an option for the Board of Examiners to omit the particular station completely and normalize the rest of the marks or make a change in the weighting of the scoring template in order to better reflect the skills to be tested.

It is imperative that the Board of Examiners carefully review the impact of the moderation exercise, including the increase or decrease of the number of students failing, before and after the moderation and to recommend how such moderation can be avoided in the future. The deliberations conducted during the moderation process must be properly documented.

Valid reasons for moderation:

- The skills tested in the OSCE did not match the learning outcomes of the curriculum or course
- The students did not get enough opportunity to practice the skills tested in the OSCE
- The OSCE marking template did not reflect what was intended in the station
- The instructions to the candidate were too ambiguous
- The simulated patients did not perform according to the scripts
- Equipment failed during the whole or a part of the OSCE

Invalid reasons for moderation:

- There are too few failures in the OSCE
- There are too many candidates with high marks
- The distribution of marks did not reach a "bell-shaped" curve

Banking of OSCE Stations

The quality assurance process also helps to identify the OSCE stations that can be stored for future usage (Ker *et al.*, 2005). When documenting a station to be banked, at the very least, the content area and the learning outcomes that the station covered, the author's name, the dates of submission, the dates of administration, the results of the item analysis for each administration, any modifications made to the station, and the item analysis results after modifications should be recorded. Below is an example of the data that can be collected in an item bank (Table 13.1). It is recommended that OSCE banking should be carried out centrally (e.g. in the Deanery, Assessment Center, or Medical Education Unit) for proper safeguarding and continuity. Banking can be done manually or electronically.

When banking a station, an electronic system using a standalone (non-networked) computer with an encrypted and password-protected security system should be employed. Each station should

Table 13.1. Example of a Data Collection Sheet for Item Banking

Basic information				Classification						Performance of the Station — First Administration				
Station Name	Date first developed	Question setters	Name of SPs	Content topics	Competencies tested	Age group	Sex	Context	Outcomes assessed (ACGME)	FI	DI	Alpha-if-item deleted*	Candidate feedback	Faculty feedback
Anxious patient	2010	AB		Mental health	Interview, history taking	20–40	F	Out-patient	Patient care, interpersonal communication skills	0.87	0.09	0.40		
Chest pain	2010	LMK	(Harvey)	Cardiovascular system	Physical examination	40–60	M	In-patient	Medical knowledge, patient care	0.92	0.15	0.37		
Inhaler use	2010	CA		Respiratory system	Patient education	40–60	M	Out-patient	Practice-based learning and improvement	0.75	0.36	0.34		

*Overall alpha reliability of the OSCE is 0.4

be tagged to the content area and learning outcomes that the station addresses, the dates of administration, and the basic categories of item parameters, so that any banked station is searchable using any of the tagged keywords or any combination of these keywords.

Summary

Quality assurance through analysis of quantitative and qualitative data helps us to identify the strengths and weaknesses of a curriculum and thereby provide us with an opportunity to improve students' learning. Feedback to the students is invaluable as a learning tool and must be a part of a good OSCE process. The post-examination review also helps us to determine whether there is any need for moderation of marks and identify OSCE stations that can be banked for future usage.

References

Branch WT, Paranjape A. (2002) Feedback and reflection: Teaching methods for clinical settings. *Acad Med* 77(12 pt 1): 1185–1188.

Ker JS, Dowie A, Dowell J, Dewar G, Dent JA, Ramsay J, Benvie S, Bracher L, Jackson C. (2005) Twelve tips for developing and maintaining a simulated patient bank. *Med Teach* 27(1): 4–9.

Khan J, Rooney K, Prosciatek C, Javadpoor A, Rooney PJ. (1997) Effect of immediate feedback on performance of subsequent stations during an objective structured clinical examination. *Educ Health* 20: 351–357.

14

HELPING POORLY PERFORMING STUDENTS IN AN OSCE

In an OSCE, students may demonstrate poor performance and may fail to achieve the expected outcomes. A properly constructed and planned OSCE program should guide examiners and faculty towards identifying poorly performing candidates. It is the responsibility of the institutes to detect underperforming students and provide them with support in order to rectify their deficiencies.

At the end of this chapter, we should be able to:

(i) Review the factors associated with the poor performance or failure of students in an OSCE.
(ii) Identify different patterns of students' failure in an OSCE.
(iii) Recognize the challenges of remediation of failed students.
(iv) Identify and delegate tasks to the right people involved in the remediation process.
(v) Develop remediation strategies and organize remediation processes for poorly performing students.

Importance of Remediation

It is ironic that the students who are most vulnerable are also those who get the least attention in the aftermath of an examination. The remediation process is often an afterthought — viewed as an extra burden of work for the faculty and examiners (Kassebaum & Eaglen,

1999; Sayer *et al.*, 2002). However, a rigorous remediation process is as important as setting up the main examination. It has to be pre-planned and built within the OSCE program. It is a legal and an ethical responsibility on the part of the institute to safeguard patients' wellbeing by detecting poor performers and applying remediation in order to achieve the expected clinical competencies among the students to the appropriate performance standards (Karen *et al.*, 2009).

Studies have shown that students' poor performance in an OSCE in earlier academic years is associated with poor performance in later academic years (Martin & Jolly, 2002). If a remediation process is not instituted properly, the problem may remain uncorrected, putting patients and students at risk. Moreover, students' poor performance in an OSCE may only be the tip of the iceberg (i.e. the surface manifestation of larger problems faced by the students). If students' learning problems are not addressed properly by the institute, there might be spillover effects on other subject areas, leading to failure in multiple subjects. Conversely, a well-developed remediation program leads to increased student satisfaction, motivates the students to achieve a higher standard of performance, and improves the pass rate in subsequent assessments (Pell *et al.*, 2012; Sayer *et al.*, 2002).

Reasons for Poor Performance in an OSCE

Students' underperformance in an examination results from several factors working either in isolation or in concert with each other. The factors could be related to the students or be a result of wider systematic issues related to the curriculum or the examination.

Before concluding that students are responsible for their poor performance, it is important to exclude factors that are not related to the students. Systematic factors, such as setting an unexpectedly high standard in the examination (see Chapter 9), wrong instructions to the candidate (see Chapter 6), discrepancies between the expected tasks and the scoring sheet (see Chapter 7), lack of examiners' standardization (see Chapter 6 and Chapter 10), and poor curricular coverage of the tested materials (see Chapter 4), are often responsible for students' underperformance in an examination. Generally speaking, a thorough evaluation of the examination, including quantitative analysis and feedback from examinees and examiners, should be sufficient for identifying wider, systematic reasons for failure (see Chapter 12). These factors are not the remit of this particular chapter. In this chapter, we will only deal with the examinee- or student-related modifiable factors that can be addressed through remediation.

Academic factors related to poor performance in an examination might be related to poor reasoning skills, improper technical skills, poor content knowledge or lack of adequate exposure to the tested materials, lack of feedback on the performance of the student (Al-Haqwi *et al.*, 2012), and unfamiliarity with the OSCE-type examination. Some of these factors may coexist or a deficiency in a given area may impact on another. For example, counseling a diabetic patient on medication safety requires adequate knowledge in the content area, as well as good communication skills. Without proper knowledge related to medication, a candidate may not be able to demonstrate the appropriate communication skills required for passing the OSCE. Academic factors are better addressed by the assigned clinical tutors or domain experts.

Stress is an important contributor to students' underperformance in an examination (Tooth, Tonge, & McManus, 1989). Although any test is an anxiety-provoking activity, the OSCE, by its nature of having direct, fast-paced, face-to-face interactions, tends to cause more anxiety and stress. Imagine a typical OSCE encounter where the students are required to perform a multitude of demanding tasks including, for example, resuscitating a collapsed patient, assessing the suicidal risk in a depressed patient, examining a patient with jaundice, breaking bad news to a cancer patient, etc. In reality, no physician is ever expected to perform such demanding tasks within an hour! Although a certain degree of stress may have a beneficial effect, excess stress is surely detrimental to the performance of the student in the examination.

Other nonacademic and personal factors that can contribute to poor performance during the examination include: Family and life difficulties; sleep deprivation prior to examination (Abdulghani *et al.*, 2012); and psychological and emotional problems. Medical education is perceived as being stressful, and a high level of stress has a negative effect on the cognitive functioning and learning of students in a medical school (Dahlin *et al.*, 2005). Nonacademic factors are better handled by the student support services, by pastoral care, and occasionally by a trained psychologist. Table 14.1 lists different factors that adversely affect student performance.

Table 14.1.   Different Factors that Adversely Affect Students' Performance

Systematic factors
- Materials not covered in the curriculum
- Lack of examiners' standardization
- A poorly developed scoring sheet
- Poorly developed instructions to the candidate

Academic factors
- Poor general academic performance
- Absenteeism
- Lack of feedback
- Unfamiliarity with the OSCE format

Nonacademic factors
- Anxiety and stress
- Family and personal issues
- Time management
- Sleep deprivation
- Lack of motivation
- Lack of proficiency in English
- Learning disabilities

The pattern of underperformance of a candidate, if apparent during the analysis, may help to identify the underlying problem (Table 14.2). A candidate may have borderline underperformance in all or most of the stations. A candidate might clearly fail in certain subject areas, such as those related to acute medicine or psychiatry, while performing well in others. He/She might demonstrate underperformance in certain competencies, such as communication or counseling, physical examination, or clinical reasoning. Finally, a random failure may have occurred, without the emergence of any specific pattern. Table 14.2 below shows potential patterns of underperformance and illustrative causes.

Table 14.2. Causes for Underperformance in an OSCE

Pattern of Underperformance	Illustrative Causes
Borderline performance in the entire OSCE	Poor academic performance, anxiety and stress, and unfamiliarity with the OSCE format
Clear failure in certain subjects	Absenteeism, lack of practice, lack of motivation in a given subject area, subjects not taught
Underperformance in certain competencies	Language barrier, general weakness in a certain competence
Multiple random failure	Multiple potential causes, which are mentioned in Table 14.1

Customization of Remediation Strategies

As the factors leading to underperformance of students in an OSCE are varied and highly specific to the individual and, to some extent, to the institute, the remediation strategy also needs to be individualized and targeted to the particular student (Hauer *et al.*, 2008; Sayer *et al.*, 2002). The process of remediation should start immediately after the OSCE is finished. It is our observation that students tend to make prior engagements and travel plans, including scheduling overseas elective rotations, before the start of the OSCE. The remediation process, if needed for a given student, may impact on these travel plans and other engagements. Therefore, students should be given sufficient advance notice that the remediation process, being an integral part of the OSCE, might be needed for certain students. Students should be advised to take note of the dates of the remediation process before making any firm commitments.

The process of remediation can be structured into four sequential steps: Referral, identifying the problems, developing a plan of actions, and retesting.

Referral

Referral of the underperforming students to the person responsible for remediation is the first crucial step. This should happen immediately after the feedback session that customarily takes place following an OSCE. The source of referral may include: Self-referral, the OSCE committee, phase committee, or any other authority responsible for students' academic wellbeing. Just like a good referral in clinical practice, the referral letter should include a brief description of the problem identified, reasons for the referral, and contact information for the person referring the students.

Identification of Problems

This is perhaps the most important step in the remediation process, akin to diagnosing a patient's problem during a clinical encounter (Sayer *et al.*, 2002). Without a proper diagnosis, the intervention will be misdirected. The encounter should start with an explanation of the purpose of the session, describing the format of the session, and the data sources to be used for the meeting. We recommend a structured meeting between the assigned faculty and the student in order to plan the process of remediation.

Identification of the causes of a student's failure includes both subjective (e.g. student's personal reflection and comments from examiners) as well as objective data (e.g. examination results). Videotaped OSCE stations, if available, provide an informative and reliable data source for identifying problem areas (Pinsky & Wipf, 2000). The available OSCE data of a student should be analyzed and discussed in the presence of the student in order to assess the deficiencies. Past performance reports, including prior performance in the OSCE, are an invaluable adjunct. Students should also learn how to assess themselves and identify their deficiencies in clinical competencies; this will enhance the skills of lifelong learning activities. If the students have difficulties in the cognitive domain, they could be instructed to enhance their knowledge by focused reading. Difficulties may be identified in specific skills, like communication, counseling, or procedural skills, which may be tackled by supervised focused practical activities (Cruess & Cruess, 2006; Papadakis *et al.*, 2005).

Students should be asked whether they would prefer the sessions to be anonymous. Similarly, prior explicit permission from the student is necessary if the session is to be audiotaped. Regardless of whether the session is audiotaped or not, detailed record keeping is essential, not only as a source of reference for the agreed plan, but also to safeguard the institution's interests in the event of possible misconduct or a complaint of mistreatment by a student in the future. The conduct of the interview should start with open-ended questions and should progressively move towards specific areas with closed-ended questions. Below is a list of questions that could be asked during the interview.

Suggested targeted questions during a remediation interview to identify the causes of failure

  (i) Where do you think the problem lies?
 (ii) Were you under undue stress during the OSCE?
(iii) Did you have a good rest or good sleep prior to the OSCE?
 (iv) Did you have any problems following the instructions in a particular station?
  (v) Was the language barrier an issue?
 (vi) Did you face similar difficulties while performing similar tasks in another situation?
(vii) Do you think the problem lies with poor knowledge or inappropriate process (e.g., way of communication) or a combination of both?
(viii) Do you have weakness in a particular area or is the problem more generic in nature?
 (ix) What can we do to help you?

Developing a Plan of Action

Once a proper cause or causes have been identified for the poor performance in the OSCE, a detailed remediation plan can be chalked out between the student and the guiding faculty. The idea is to have a negotiated plan of action with progressive empowerment of the student and shared responsibility between the student and the faculty. The student should take ownership of the problem and should be guided to achieve specific goals. The plan of action should have specific targets and deliverables, detail the frequency and duration of engagement, plan for an interim evaluation in order to judge the progress made so far, and provide a mock mini-OSCE, if needed.

Plan of action

(i) Generate specific and targeted learning objectives
(ii) Detail the frequency and duration of engagement
(iii) Suggest a date of mid-term evaluation
(iv) Ensure student self-assessment of the progress
(v) Provide a mock mini-OSCE

These activities have to be designed in such a way that they fulfill the individual underperforming student's needs. As the remediation process is a difficult and time-consuming, enthusiastic clinical tutors need to be selected to take part in the remediation process. These tutors should have good academic records and should also be popular among the students. For academic causes of poor performance, all forms of teaching and learning activities can be utilized, based on the individual needs assessment. For example, the student may require extra clinical training in ambulatory care clinics with real patients, standardized patients (SPs) and mannequins in a skills laboratory for specific procedural skills, or an extra placement in specific subject areas. As the basic tenet of a remediation process is the improvement and support of the student, tutor and SP feedback should be essential elements of the remediation process (Ericsson,

2004). Sufficient practice should be allowed for the remediation process, based on the availability of the candidates' time and teaching resources. For many nonacademic causes of poor performance, it might be necessary to seek help from the Deanship of Student Affairs and other student support services that are available within the institute. Finally, a workable plan needs to be devised for the identified problems, remediation actions, and responsibility. An example of such a plan is shown below (Table 14.3).

Table 14.3. Possible Specific Strategies for Specific Problems Identified During Remediation

Problem	Remediation	Responsibility
Difficulties in following instructions in the OSCE; poor command of English	Remedial sessions in English for this specific purpose; self-practice with an audio-tape	Examinee English tutor
Poor time management; cramming before the examination	Time management strategies; specific targeted learning before the examination	Mentor
Living away from campus (e.g. drives 90 min each way)	Arrange in-campus accommodation	Student housing
Poor techniques in neurological examination	Extra tutorial on neurological examination with patients	Clinical tutor
Inadequate exposure to emergency patient encounters	Extra sessions with simulation	Clinical tutor

Retesting of the Candidates After Remediation

Retesting after remediation must be equivalent to the main examination in the form of content coverage, task representation, difficulty level, and pass/fail criteria. The retesting can take place in the form of either a full-scale OSCE (e.g. if the student failed in multiple random stations and there is no specific pattern of deficiencies) or a more focused OSCE in particular domains where the candidate failed (e.g. if a candidate failed only in procedural skills, a procedural skill-focused OSCE is an alternative to a full-scale OSCE). Often, such a decision is based on the number of failed candidates, faculty resources, and whether the OSCE is high stakes or medium stakes in nature. As the remediation is an important component of the learning process, sufficient time should be allocated between the main examination and the retesting. A retesting that appears soon after the main examination can be legitimately questioned as to whether the time provided was sufficient for the student to learn and remediate.

Challenges in Remediation

Remediation is costly in terms of student and faculty time. The extra workload involved in the remediation process may produce psychological effects on the students and faculty. Continuous formative assessment and feedback to trainees may reduce the burden of remediation. A mock OSCE can be beneficial for learning clinical skills and may reduce the failure rate. Finally, a well-developed educational program should have sufficient checks in place to identify potentially poorly performing students early in the course and should provide longitudinal guidance throughout. This will reduce the burden of the remediation exercise after an OSCE.

Summary

Remediation of underperforming students is an important and integral part of a good assessment system. Essential elements of a successful remediation process include identifying the problems of students who need remediation using multiple data sources and developing an individualized learning plan by providing instructions that include deliberate practice, feedback, reflection, reassessment, and certification of competence. Remediation is a shared and collaborative process with progressive responsibility delegated to the students during the period of remediation.

References

Abdulghani HM, Alrowais NA, Bin-Saad NS, Al-Subaie NM, Haji AM, Al-Haqwi AI. (2012) Sleep disorder among medical students: Relationship to their academic performance. *Med Teach* **34**: S37–S41.

Al-Haqwi AI, Al-Wahbi A, Abdulghani HM, van der Molen TH, Schmidt HG. (2012) Barriers of feedback in undergraduate medical education in Saudi Arabia. *Saudi Med J* **33**(5): 179–183.

Cruess RL, Cruess SR. (2006) Teaching professionalism: General principles. *Med Teach* **28**(3): 205–208.

Ericsson KA. (2004) Deliberate practice and the acquisition and maintenance of expert performance in medicine and related domains. *Acad Med* **79**(10 suppl.): S70–S81.

Hauer KE, Ciccone A, Henzel TR, Katsufrakis P, Miller SH, Norcross WA, Papadakis MA, Irby DM. (2009) Remediation of the deficiencies of physicians across the continuum from medical school to practice: A thematic review of the literature. *Acad Med* **84**(12): 1822–1832.

Hauer KE, Teherani A, Irby DM, Kerr KM, O'Sullivan PS. (2008) Approaches to medical student remediation after a comprehensive clinical skills examination. *Med Educ* **42**(1): 104–112.

Kassebaum DG, Eaglen RH. (1999) Shortcomings in the evaluation of students clinical skills and behaviors in medical school. *Acad Med* **74**(7): 842–849.

Papadakis MA, Teherani A, Banach MA, Knetller TR, Rattner SL, Stern DT, Veloski JJ, Hodgson CS. (2005) Disciplinary action by medical boards and prior behavior in medical school. *N Engl J Med* **353**(25): 2673–2682.

Pell G, Fuller R, Homer M, Roberts T. (2012) Is short-term remediation after OSCE failure sustained? A retrospective analysis of the longitudinal attainment of underperforming students in OSCE assessments. *Med Teach* **34**(2): 146–150.

Pinsky L, Wipf J. (2000). A picture is worth a thousand words: Practical use of videotape in teaching. *J Gen Intern Med* **15**(11): 805–810.

Sayer M, Saintonge MC, Evans D, Wood D. (2002) Support for students with academic difficulties. *Med Educ* **36**(7): 643–650.

Tooth D, Tonge K, McManus IC. (1989) Anxiety and study methods in preclinical students: Causal relation to academic performance. *Med Educ* **23**(5): 416–421.

15

OSCE AS A TOOL FOR THE SELECTION OF APPLICANTS

The OSCE format can be used not only for the assessment of clinical skills in the conventional, end-of-course context, but also for the assessment of behavior (i.e. both skills and attitudes) in general in varied contexts. To illustrate such a utilization of the OSCE in different contexts, this chapter details the adaptation of the OSCE format for the development of a selection tool to admit applicants to healthcare education courses.

At the end of this chapter, we should be able to:

(i) Recognize the flexibility of the OSCE format for catering to different assessment purposes, such as the selection of applicants to healthcare education courses.

(ii) Utilize the OSCE format to assess aptitude (i.e. in the context of selection), as opposed to competence, regarding technical skills.

(iii) Identify the strengths and the limitations of the OSCE when used for selection purposes.

(iv) Evaluate the utility of a selection OSCE when combined with the other selection tools.

The Flexibility of the OSCE Format

It is well known that the OSCE was initially devised to assess the clinical skills of medical students (Harden *et al.*, 1975). However, of late, the OSCE format has been used in different contexts, whenever there has been a need to assess the ability of the candidate through a sample of standardized, simulated situations. Two related examples of the use of the OSCE format in the context of the selection of applicants to healthcare education courses are the Selection OSCE (Ponnamperuma, 2009) and the Multiple Mini-Interview (MMI) (Eva *et al.*, 2004a).

These two tools are similar to the extent that both assess candidates' aptitude, using multiple hypothetical situations, in relation to the generic competencies that are necessary to study in a healthcare education course, as well as to be a good healthcare professional in the future. The competencies that are commonly assessed by both of these tools are communication skills, teamwork and leadership, reasoning skills, ability to respond to challenging situations, ethics, attitudes, and professionalism.

However, the two tools do have a fundamental difference. The MMI uses the "oral examination" as its base, while the Selection OSCE is based on the classical OSCE format (i.e. enacted simulated situations). So, in the typical MMI, the oral examiner asks the candidate a few predetermined questions on a certain theme (e.g. abortion), as they would ask in a structured oral examination. Such questions may often be based on a hypothetical scenario that is given to the candidate before the examiner starts their questioning. The oral examiner then scores the candidate's oral answers using an objective and structured assessment instrument, such as a rating scale or a checklist. However, in a Selection OSCE that uses enacted hypothetical situations, the candidate has to interact with a simulated person (i.e. not necessarily a simulated patient), as the situations are more generic, everyday situations, rather than healthcare-related situations. Such an interaction is observed and objectively scored (as in a classical OSCE), using the same scoring instruments as discussed earlier (i.e. rating scales and checklists) by an examiner. In this sense, the Selection OSCE samples the candidate's behavior in a more authentic (i.e. real-life) manner when compared with the oral examination in the MMI. Hence, it is argued that the candidate's chances of being able to fake a given competency is reduced in the Selection OSCE, as the candidate needs to enact their response to a given situation, rather than orally stating what they would do in a given situation (Ponnamperuma, 2009).

That being said, the MMI has recently been modified to benefit from the advantages of the OSCE format. The main advantage of the modified MMI is the inclusion of some stations that have simulated persons or at least the examiner acting as a simulated person. This could be viewed as a hybrid version that combines the features of the Selection OSCE and the MMI.

How to Develop a Selection OSCE

The following are the steps for developing a selection OSCE:

(i) Decide on the competencies to be assessed. The competency framework (i.e. the exit learning outcomes) of the course to which the candidates are selected should be the competency framework from which the competencies should be selected for the Selection OSCE. In fact, any selection test should be viewed as the first assessment of the battery of assessments of a healthcare education course. However, in using the competency framework of the healthcare education course, there are a few caveats:

  (a) All of the exit learning outcomes of the course may not be suitable for a selection test. For example, outcomes such as clinical skills cannot be assessed at selection (except in postgraduate selection). Hence, the outcomes that can be tested should only be selected for a Selection OSCE.

  (b) Some outcomes, such as procedural skills, cannot be assessed to the same extent as in an actual in-course or end-of-course OSCE, since the candidates will not have taken a formal course on these outcomes. Therefore, only the underlying principle(s) that underpins the performance of a given procedural skill can be assessed in a Selection OSCE. For example, venepuncture cannot be assessed in a Selection OSCE that selects candidates for an undergraduate medical course. However, the *principle* that underpins the successful performance of venepuncture, which is "hand-eye coordination," can be assessed using a video game.

(c) The level at which the selected outcomes need to be tested is at the level of "aptitude." That is, the level of assessment should be to determine the *potential* of the candidate to achieve the assessed exit learning outcomes during a formal educational program, rather than the achievement of the said outcomes per se. The latter can be only tested at the end of a formal educational program, and not at the stage of selection to an educational program.

(ii) Select the contents through which the above competencies or outcomes will be assessed. When selecting content, since there is no specified curriculum or a list of topics (i.e. a syllabus), especially in undergraduate selection, one has to consider the generic, everyday activities or scenarios that a typical applicant would encounter. These scenarios could be modelled according to "situational judgment tests," which have been extensively used for personnel selection for employment in general (McDaniel *et al.*, 2001). For example, advising a friend or discussing a confidential issue with a friend could be taken as the content material based on which outcomes such as communication skills, ethics, attitudes, and professionalism are tested. At least 10 such stations should be included, with each station lasting for about 5–10 minutes.

(iii) Develop a selection blueprint as discussed in the previous chapters, by meshing the competencies (Step i) with the content scenarios (Step ii) identified above. Knowledge-related (i.e. cognitive) outcomes, such as "basic and social sciences knowledge," should not be assessed as the only outcomes tested within a given scenario. Rather, such knowledge-related outcomes should be tested as auxiliary outcomes, along with other behavior-related outcomes, which should be the predominant outcomes for a given Selection OSCE station. In general, as discussed previously, any scenario should assess a combination of outcomes, rather than one outcome (i.e. as in any other OSCE, the Selection OSCE should also contain "integrated stations").

(iv) As discussed in previous chapters, once the selection blueprint is designed, convert the identified scenario content within each station into a proper OSCE station by developing the candidate instructions, the examiner instructions along with the necessary rating scales and checklists, the simulated person instructions, and a list of equipment, together with any other instructions that are necessary to implement the station. A station developed this way is given in Appendix 15.1 as an illustration.

(v) Train the examiners and the simulated persons (i.e. the actors). Each station should be manned by a trained examiner, usually a staff member who teaches the course (i.e. educational program) to which the candidates are selected. On special occasions, other trained examiners can also be employed. However, the advantage of having teachers as examiners is that they can readily visualize the characteristics of a candidate who is suitable to follow the course. When training examiners, special attention should be paid to impress upon the examiners that they should use the checklists and the rating scales in order to assess the *potential* of the candidates in achieving the learning outcomes, rather than the actual achievement of the said outcomes.

(vi) Pilot the Selection OSCE and, based on the pilot results, make the necessary changes, where applicable.

(vii) Usually criterion-referenced standard setting is not carried out for selection tests, as selecting the highest scorers using norm referencing is the accepted practice. However, in order to prevent selection of candidates who have scored unacceptably poorly in one competency (across all stations), but have compensated for such poor performance by scoring well in other competencies, one could set a minimum threshold for each competency before applying norm referencing to the Selection OSCE. Such an approach would prevent excessive compensation among competencies.

(viii) Implement the Selection OSCE and evaluate its utility, as discussed in the following sections.

Evaluating the Utility of the Selection OSCE

When evaluating the utility of the Selection OSCE, the criteria similar to those used in previous chapters could be used (i.e. reliability, validity, acceptability, educational impact, and practicality (feasibility and cost-effectiveness)). Out of these criteria, there is satisfactory evidence on acceptability, especially with regards to the candidates and examiners (Humphrey *et al.*, 2008). Although specific studies on educational impact, practicability, and feasibility are relatively rare, the few studies published so far (Rosenfeld *et al.*, 2008) and the widespread adoption of the MMI indicate that the issues related to these criteria are certainly surmountable, especially given the wealth of information that the MMI provides about the candidate. With regards to reliability, studies in relation to both the MMI and the Selection OSCE indicate that approximately 10 stations with live, simulated encounters would provide acceptable reliability.

With regards to validity, content validity could be easily achieved through a blueprint designed as detailed in this chapter. However, the most important form of validity that one should investigate is predictive validity. Studies in relation to both the MMI (Eva *et al.*, 2004b) and the Selection OSCE (Ponnamperuma, 2009) have found them to have acceptable predictive validity, especially with regards to the ability of the MMI/Selection OSCE to predict behavior-related competencies (Ponnamperuma, 2009; Reiter *et al.*, 2007).

Strengths and Limitations of the Selection OSCE

The Selection OSCE is designed to benefit from the undisputed advantages of the OSCE format; that is, the ability to assess a candidate by exposing him or her to a wide sample of test material (i.e. practical situations) and examiners. Such a format enables the assessment of competencies that cannot be assessed objectively using traditional selection tests.

However, the Selection OSCE only assesses the candidate's behavior and thereby the candidate's potential to be trained into an appropriate professional. It does not assess the candidate's behavior in real situations; it only assesses the candidate at the "Shows how" level of Miller's pyramid, and not at the "Does" level. The Selection OSCE also does not directly assess a candidate's cognitive ability. As such, the results of the Selection OSCE should be combined with other appropriate selection measures, such as the results of previous written examinations and written aptitude tests.

Summary

The Selection OSCE is a selection method that capitalizes on the sampling ability of the OSCE to select the most suitable candidates for educational courses by assessing their aptitude/potential to achieve the learning outcomes of the course (especially the learning outcomes related to behavior), using multiple (i.e. a wide sample of) practical, simulated situations and examiners. The MMI also uses the OSCE format to expose candidates to a wide sample of situations and examiners. However, classically, the MMI is based on oral assessment, whereas the Selection OSCE is firmly based on the OSCE format that assesses hands-on skills, using live, simulated situations. Thus, the candidate's chances of being able to fake a given competency in relation to the Selection OSCE is arguably reduced when compared with the oral examination format. Hence, recent MMIs have included OSCE-type stations in order to assess the candidate's actual ability (not only the spoken ability, as assessed in the oral examination format) in simulated, live situations.

The Selection OSCE, which has approximately 10 properly blueprinted stations, with each station manned by a single examiner, has demonstrated acceptable reliability and predictive validity regarding the candidate's future performance, especially in behavior-related competencies. As the Selection OSCE tests the candidate only at "Shows how" level, results from the Selection OSCE should be combined with other acceptable selection parameters, such as the candidate's previous written examination results, in order to select the most appropriate candidates.

References

Eva KW, Rosenfeld J, Reiter HI, Norman GR. (2004a) An admissions OSCE: The Multiple Mini-Interview. *Med Educ* **38**(3): 314–326.

Eva KW, Reiter HI, Rosenfeld J, Norman GR. (2004b) The ability of the Multiple Mini-Interview to predict pre-clerkship performance in medical school. *Acad Med* **79**(10 suppl.): S40–S42.

Harden RM, Stevenson M, Downie WW, Wilson GM. (1975) Assessment of clinical competence using objective structured examination. *Br Med J* **1**(5955): 447–451.

Humphrey S, Dowson S, Wall D, Diwakar V, Goodyear HM. (2008) Multiple mini-interviews: Opinions of candidates and interviewers. *Med Educ* **42**(2): 207–213.

McDaniel MA, Morgeson FP, Finnegan EB, Campion MA, Braverman EP. (2001) Use of situational judgment tests to predict job performance: A clarification of the literature. *J Appl Psychol* **86**(4): 730–740.

Ponnamperuma G. (2009) *Medical School Selection: A Competency-based Approach*. VDM Verlag, Germany.

Reiter HI, Eva KW, Rosenfeld J, Norman GR. (2007) Multiple mini-interviews predict clerkship and licensing examination performance. *Med Educ* **41**(4): 378–384.

Rosenfeld JM, Reiter HI, Trinh K, Eva KW. (2008) A cost efficiency comparison between the multiple mini-interview and traditional admissions interviews. *Adv Health Sci Educ Theory Pract* **13**(1): 43–58.

APPENDIX 15.1: AN EXAMPLE OF A SELECTION OSCE STATION

Instructions to the Candidate

You borrowed a book from a friend to study for the examination. The friend gave this book to you with the understanding that he will receive the book in time for him to study for the same examination. However, now you cannot find the book (i.e. you have misplaced the book). There is only one more week before the examination and the friend has asked for the book from you. Talk to your friend regarding this issue.

Station time: 5 min.

Instructions to the Simulated Friend

You have to act in this station as a friend of the candidate. You lent a textbook that is essential for you to study for the examination to this friend of yours with the agreement that he/she will return the book in time for you to study for the examination. Now there is only one more week before the examination and you have asked for the book from your friend. Your friend has misplaced the book. You have now met the friend and want to know why he/she has not returned the book.

First, respond to the greetings of the candidate appropriately. For example, you could respond, "Thanks, I am well," if the candidate asks, "Hi, how are you?"

After the initial greetings, ask: "I wonder whether you could return the book that you borrowed, as I need it to study for my exam. As you know, there is just one more week before the exam."

If the candidate does not say that he/she has lost/misplaced the book, demand angrily that the book be returned immediately.

If the candidate says that he/she has misplaced the book and apologizes for it, show your disappointment. Also say that you never expected such irresponsible and unprofessional behavior from him/her.

If the candidate apologizes and says that he/she will find you another book (from the library or from some other source) without delay, then look satisfied with such a suggestion.

At the end of the station, before the next candidate arrives, please mark the most appropriate box based on the conversation that you had with the candidate.

Description of Your Feeling/Decision	Tick Box	Marks
I feel dejected for associating with a friend like this.		0
I understand that this has been a genuine lapse of an otherwise responsible friend. We will continue to be friends, but I will not lend any of my belongings to him/her again.		3
I understand that this has been a genuine lapse of an otherwise responsible friend. We will continue to be friends, and I will lend any of my belongings to him/her again, if the necessity arises.		6

Instructions to the Examiner

In this Selection OSCE station, you are expected to assess the candidate's *potential* to be developed into an honest, responsible, and professional healthcare professional who can empathize with another person's feelings and can communicate convincingly and confidently even during demanding and stressful situations. Hence, the outcomes assessed in this station are professionalism, ethics and attitudes, communication skills, and decision-making ability (or creativity).

The following is the marking checklist, in two parts (Part A and Part B). In Part A, please tick the most appropriate box (only one box) based on the candidate's behavior that you observed. Please go through the instructions to the candidate and simulated friend before reading the examiner's instruction.

Action	Tick Box	Marks
Does not say that he/she has misplaced the book. Tries to evade the issue.		0
Tells the friend that he/she has misplaced book, and gives flimsy reasons for misplacing the book (i.e. candidate does not want to accept responsibility).		2
Tells the friend that he/she has misplaced the book, but says nothing beyond this.		4
Tells the friend that he/she has misplaced the book, and unconditionally apologizes or accepts full responsibility.		6
Comes up with an alternative solution (e.g. borrowing another book from the library or from another source) so that the friend does not lose out.		8
Comes up with an alternative solution, with a definitive time scale, given the urgency of the situation.		10

In Part B, tick all of relevant boxes that you consider to be appropriate for the observed behavior of the candidate.

Checklist Item	Tick Box	Marks
Communicates in a mood that is appropriate for the situation.		2
Empathizes with the disappointment of the friend.		2
Expresses his/her own disappointment about his/her own lapse.		2
Communicates clearly and confidently the solution that is proposed, gaining the confidence (rather than the suspicion) of the friend.		2
Consoles the friend in a reassuring manner (e.g. "Don't worry. I will not allow you to be at a disadvantage").		2

Part C is the global rating scale. In Part C, please mark the appropriate box in order to indicate your impressions about the candidate's overall ability. Please mark this independently of the checklist items that you marked in Parts A and B.

0	1	2	3	4

Very poor   Excellent

List of Equipment

✓ Candidate instructions sheet pasted on the wall and the table.
✓ Marking sheets for the examiner.
✓ Marking sheets for the simulated friend.
✓ Three chairs. Two arranged face-to-face for the simulated friend and the candidate, and the other for the examiner placed in one corner of the room so that the candidate's facial expressions can be clearly seen.

16

FREQUENTLY ASKED QUESTIONS ABOUT THE OSCE

This chapter is devoted to the compilation of frequently asked questions regarding the OSCE. The answers provided are based on contemporary evidence and best practices coupled with our collective judgment.

What is the Optimum Number of Stations in an OSCE?

The reliability of an OSCE is a function of its number of stations. It is imperative that there is a sufficient number of stations representing a range of clinical skills in an OSCE. In order to ensure content validity, a carefully developed blueprint provides a concrete guide to the number of stations needed to sample the curriculum adequately. Although reliability and validity depend on many factors, and hence a proper psychometric analysis is needed to come to a defensible answer, at least 12–16 stations are in general considered adequate to reach acceptable reliability.

What Should be the Length of Each Station?

The length of station depends on the nature of the task to be completed in a given station. However, for practical reasons, all OSCE stations are allocated the same duration (exception: long-station OSCEs or double stations). Although an OSCE station typically represents only a part of the consultation process, a useful gauge is to consider the time taken to conduct a consultation in the health-care setting. Typically, an out-patient consultation lasts 10–15 min. You should also remember to factor in the time taken for the candidate to move from one station to another, the time required to read the instructions to the candidate, and time for the examiners to mark the station. One should also keep in mind the trade-off between the duration of time per station and the number of stations. The longer the station, the lesser the number of stations that could be included in the OSCE. Reducing the number of stations by increasing the station duration will adversely affect the content validity and reliability of the OSCE. So, the goal should be to optimize the duration per station without compromising the number of stations included in the OSCE.

Should there be Two Examiners per Station or One Examiner per Station?

Having two examiners per station provides marginal additional benefit to the reliability of an OSCE station over having one examiner per station. Although the inter-rater reliability between the two examiners marking the same station tends to be high, this is often due to collusion between the examiners. Hence, it is preferable to allocate one examiner per station and increase the number of stations instead. This will have a greater impact on the reliability (and validity, especially content validity) of the examination.

Can We have an OSCE with Variable Durations of Stations?

Yes, it is possible to have OSCE stations of variable durations within the same circuit. However, the long stations' durations need to be multiples of the short stations' durations. For example, if a short station's duration is 10 minutes, the long stations' durations need to be 20 minutes or 30 minutes. In other words, the long stations cannot be 15 minutes in duration.

Do We Need to have a Rest Station in an OSCE?

Rest stations, where a candidate is not required to perform any task, provide the candidate with a well-deserved break during the OSCE. It is our recommendation to include a rest station for an OSCE that has more than 10 stations or that is more than 120 min in duration. Be mindful that a rest station is most beneficial to candidates who are in the middle of the circuit. A rest station is less useful for the candidate who starts the OSCE with a rest station and the candidate who ends the OSCE with a rest station. Rest can also be provided by having one or two shorter OSCE stations in which the task can be completed before the allocated time. We also suggest that if the candidate completes the task before the allocated time, they should be allowed to step out of the room. This will allow the candidate, examiners, and patients to take a break.

Do We Need Expert Examiners for an OSCE?

It depends on the nature of the task to be tested in the examination. For an OSCE that tests clinical judgments and medical decision-making, it is necessary to have content experts as examiners. For simpler tasks or procedures, trained non-expert examiners are sufficient. Moreover, the definition of "expert" is also open to interpretation. For example, for an OSCE station testing a normal cardiovascular examination, an expert could be defined as a general physician or an internist or a cardiologist. For simplicity, the expertise required from the experts should match the tasks to be performed by the examinee, and reducing the reliance on expert examiners is entirely plausible in many OSCE stations.

Can We Include Non-Physicians as OSCE Examiners?

Absolutely, many tasks that physicians are required to perform and are tested in an OSCE do not need physicians as examiners. It might be argued that, for certain tasks, non-physicians such as nurses are better suited as examiners. Examples of such tasks include skills stations such as intravenous catheter insertion, patient education stations such as teaching patients the correct way of injecting insulin, and counseling and communication stations such as handover of patients.

Should the Patient Mark the OSCE Station?

It is possible for *well-trained* standardized patients and simulated patients to mark the candidate during the OSCE. It makes sense to have the patients mark the candidate, particularly on elements related to communication and professionalism. However, this adds to the cognitive load of the standardized or simulated patients and this may negatively impact on their performance.

Should the Examiners Provide Feedback to the Candidate during the OSCE?

Feedback to the candidate is an integral component of any good assessment practice. However, in a high-stakes summative OSCE, we do not recommend giving feedback while the OSCE is in motion. In a highly pressurized examination situation, neither the examiner nor the candidate is in a position to provide or receive feedback, respectively. Furthermore, negative feedback may upset the candidate, leading to adverse performance in the subsequent stations. Instead, our recommendation is to note down qualitative comments about the candidate's performance during the OSCE and provide the candidate with the feedback after the OSCE.

Should the Examiners Ask Questions of the Candidate during the OSCE?

Generally speaking, for the vast majority of the tasks that are tested in an OSCE, marking is based on checklists or rating scales. There is no need for the examiners to ask questions during the OSCE. However, for certain tasks, especially those related to clinical judgments and decision-making, it might be necessary for the examiners to ask a few selected questions in order to assess the candidate's interpretative, judgmental, or decision-making skills. It is imperative that such questions are predetermined and model answers are provided to the examiners. Alternatively, the candidates could write down their findings after completing the interactions with the patients for them to be marked later.

Can We have Real Patients in an OSCE?

Yes, certain tasks can only be realistically tested with real patients. Examples of such tasks could be edema, joint swellings, and other fixed abnormalities. However, real patient needs to be properly trained and briefed in order to minimize variability. In other words, real patients need to be standardized. An alternative to real patients are simulated patients or trained lay persons portraying a given medical condition.

Can We Use Clinical Photographs in an OSCE?

Clinical materials, including audiovisual recordings, X-rays, and pathological specimens, can be successfully incorporated into the OSCE. If used, they should be integrated with patient scenarios. For example, the findings obtained during a colonoscopy can be incorporated with a scenario of a patient presenting with altered bowel movement. However, all of these stations should involve some tasks to be performed by the candidate that cannot be tested using a written or computer-based assessment. The stations should not be testing only knowledge, which can be tested easily through much less labor-intensive written/computer-based examinations.

Should there be Any "Killer" Stations in an OSCE?

A "killer" station is a station that a candidate must pass before passing the OSCE overall. In other words, if he/she passes all or most of the other stations, but fails in the killer station, he/she then fails in the OSCE overall. Frequently, such stations are deemed to be critical for the practice of medicine. We recommend testing these tasks separately, similar to the way competence in Basic Cardiac Life Support (BCLS) or Advance Cardiac Life Support (ACLS) is certified. There should *not* be any killer stations in an OSCE.

Can We have Two OSCE Stations that are Linked Together?

Yes, in some situations it might be desirable to have two consecutive stations that are linked together. Such stations might include tasks that are too lengthy to complete in one OSCE station and tasks that can be logically linked together. For example, in the first station, the candidate is asked to take a history and perform a physical examination on a given patient. In the second station, he/she is required to explain the findings to the patient. However, we do not recommend using too many linked stations, as this restricts the number of content areas that can be tested in a given OSCE.

Which One of the Two Marking Methods, Checklist or Rating, is Superior?

A checklist item could be used to indicate whether a certain step or action was conducted during the OSCE. However, it cannot indicate the level at which this step/action was conducted. This means checklists score the candidate's behavior in an all-or-none manner. In contrast, rating scales can be used to *grade* the candidate's behavior in order to indicate the level at which such behavior took place. Hence, checklists and rating scales have relative advantages and disadvantages. Psychometrically speaking, both methods of marking provide almost equivalent reliability, although some recent studies point to the superiority of global rating scales over checklists. However, a checklist is essential when non-expert examiners are used in the OSCE. Checklists are also useful for providing feedback to the candidate at the end of the OSCE. Global ratings, on the other hand, are useful for getting an overall impression of the candidate. In addition, ratings in general are useful for assessing competencies that are, by nature, more qualitative than quantitative (e.g. communication skills and professionalism). These are elements of competency that are not effectively captured by a checklist. In a summative OSCE, it is our recommendation to use both checklists as well as global ratings.

How Many Items Should a Checklist Contain?

It depends on the nature of the tasks to be performed during the OSCE. Some tasks by their inherent nature need a longer checklist, while for others a shorter checklist is sufficient. The length of a checklist also depends on whether one wants to lump or split elements of the tasks. Nevertheless, a too-lengthy checklist is cumbersome to complete and imposes unnecessary cognitive load on the examiners. Conversely, too short a checklist leaves room for subjective interpretation and guessing. Therefore, our recommendation is to keep the number of items in a checklist to around 10–15.

How Can We Determine the Pass/Fail Mark of the OSCE?

The pass/fail mark of the OSCE should not be based on an arbitrary standard, such as 50% or 60%. The complexity of the tasks and expectations from the candidates vary considerably from one OSCE to another. Therefore, the pass/fail boundary should also vary from one OSCE to another. The process of determining the pass/fail boundary is known as standard setting, for which there are several available methods. We recommend the borderline regression method for determining the pass/fail score in an OSCE.

How Do We Maintain Examination Security when there are Multiple Sessions?

If you have a lot of candidates to test, it might not be possible to complete the examining of all of the candidates through multiple parallel circuits within a single session. In such situations, you have to run the OSCE at least twice. Candidates who have just completed the OSCE need to be quarantined and segregated carefully until the second session's candidates start their OSCE. If there are three sessions, the first session's candidates need to be quarantined during the second session all the way through to the beginning of the third session. The second session's candidates need to be quarantined until the third session begins. Candidates should not have any access to mobile phones or computers. We recommend utilizing the quarantined time to collect feedback from the candidates about the OSCE that they have already completed.

How Should We Select a Venue for the OSCE?

Selecting a suitable venue for an OSCE can be challenging. Few medical schools are equipped with dedicated examination centers with a sufficient number of rooms that can be used for the OSCE. Hospital wards are seldom useful as OSCE venues because of frequent distractions and the absence of sound barriers. Possible venues for an OSCE could be tutorial rooms or unused clinics. We suggest using clinic rooms during the weekend for a large-scale OSCE. An alternative could be a large hall, which can be converted into multiple cubicles/rooms on a temporary basis.

How Can We Run an OSCE Over Two Days?

For logistical reasons, it might be necessary to run multiple OSCE sessions over two days. You need to prepare two sets of OSCE questions, examiners, patients, and all support staff. It is extremely important to develop the blueprint and the stations carefully, so that the OSCE on the first day is similar to, but not the same as, the second day's OSCE in terms of the breadth of content covered and the difficulty of test material.

Can We Videotape OSCE Stations?

Videotaping, if such a facility is available, is an excellent option for a high-quality OSCE. Recorded videotapes of candidates during an OSCE can be used for standardized marking, quality assurance (e.g., uncovering potential examiner biases, potential standardized patient biases, and differences in examiner stringency), and feedback purposes. Videotapes can also be preserved for future records, in case of potential disputes or complaints by the candidates. They could be further utilized for remediation purposes. Videotaping needs to be carried out unobtrusively and with prior permission from the candidate.

How Much Time do We Need to Prepare for an OSCE?

A high-quality OSCE needs careful planning, preparation, trial running, revision, and implementation. For a high-stakes summative OSCE, such as an exit-level OSCE or a year-end promotion OSCE, we recommend that the process should start 6–9 months in advance. For an end-of-rotation OSCE, the recommended preparation time is approximately 2 months.

INDEX

Absolute standard, 136
Acceptability, 23, 24, 33, 34, 101
Active station, 56, 61
Actors, 6, 68, 95, 104, 181
Alpha if item deleted, 147, 148, 153
Angoff method, 136
Arbitrary standard, 195
Authenticity, viii, 11, 83, 94–96, 113, 119

Banking of OSCE station, 158, 159, 162
Basic sciences, 42, 43, 45–48, 61, 62
Behavior, 10, 11, 18, 30, 31, 33, 42, 43, 45–48, 70, 73, 80, 86, 98, 160, 177, 178, 181–184, 186, 187, 194
Blueprint, v, vi, 25, 32, 33, 37–42, 44, 45, 49–52, 54, 65, 75, 101, 106, 122, 180, 181, 182, 189, 196
Borderline candidate, 136, 137, 140

Borderline regression method, 89, 133, 140–142, 195
Briefing of examiners, 103
Briefing of patients, 102

Checklist, vi, 4, 15, 16, 21, 32, 65, 71, 76–83, 85–87, 89, 90, 96, 124, 129, 131, 137, 139–141, 178, 181, 186, 188, 192, 194, 195
Classical borderline group method, 137, 140, 141
Cognition, 7, 10, 110
Compensatory standard, 138, 142
Conjunctive standard, 138, 142
Content expert, 81, 103, 105, 191
Content validity, 19, 21, 24, 26, 30, 34, 37, 38, 54, 182, 189, 190
Context specificity, 17
Cost, 23, 34
Couplet station, 58
Cronbach alpha, 147

Diagonal sampling, 28, 30, 31
Difficulty index, 144
Direct Observation of
  Procedural Skills, 11
Discriminatory index, 86
Does level, 11, 12, 18, 20, 94,
  183
Double station, 59, 67, 189

Educational impact, 23, 24, 30,
  32, 34, 77, 122, 182
Equipment and materials
  73–75
Examinee-centered standard
  setting, 142

Face validity, 33
Facility index, 144, 145, 148,
  153
Faculty training, xi, 89, 101,
  121–123
Fail, vii, 3, 33, 78, 80, 81, 84,
  85, 133–135, 148, 165, 168,
  173, 193, 195
False fail, 134
False pass, 134
Feasibility, 24, 128, 182
Feedback, viii, 11, 17, 32, 33,
  56, 69, 72, 78, 86, 89,
  103–105, 111, 125, 127,
  143, 144, 154–159, 159,
  160, 163, 164, 167, 168,
  170, 172, 174, 192, 194,
  196, 197
Formative OSCE, 55, 56

Generic marking template, 87,
  88

Global marking, 32, 81, 89,
  90

Harden, RM, 2-5, 7, 9, 10, 93,
  96, 177,
Harvey, 74, 113, 163
Holistic assessment, 9
Human Patient Simulator
  (HPS), 113
Hybrid simulation, 110, 116

Instructions for examiners 27,
  66, 71, 72, 76
Instructions for students, 71
Item analysis, 143, 144, 153,
  162
Itemized marking, 32, 56, 87,
  89, 90, 103

Knowledge, viii, xi, 6, 10, 11,
  12, 19, 61, 62, 90, 122, 124,
  160, 163, 167, 171, 180,
  181, 193

Linked station, 58, 59, 63, 83,
  194
Long case, 2, 3, 15, 128
Long station, 59, 63, 189,
  190

Mannequin, 5, 6, 19, 31, 71,
  73, 74, 84, 93–96, 98,
  99, 105, 110, 113–118,
  172
Master blueprint, 37, 40–42,
  44, 54, 65, 122
Miller's pyramid, 9, 10, 18, 20,
  21, 94, 183

Mini Clinical Evaluation Exercise (mini-CEX), 9, 94
Moderation of mark, 158, 159, 161, 164
Multiple choice questions, 3
Multiple Mini-Interview (MMI), 178
Multisource feedback (MSF), 11

National Board of Medical Examiners (NBME), 123

OSCE pretenders, 9, 19
OSCE team, 159
OSPE, 60, 61

PACES, 87
Pass, vii, xviii, 3, 16, 33, 38, 71, 78, 83, 86, 88, 125, 128, 133–138, 140, 141, 145, 148, 166, 173, 193, 195
Performance, v, viii, 5, 11, 12, 32, 69, 78, 80, 81, 85–87, 90, 93, 94, 116, 124, 125, 135, 144, 159, 160, 163, 165–170, 172, 173, 179, 180, 184, 192
Pilot run, 127, 128
Point biserial, 146
Post-assessment quality assurance, 143
Programmed patient, 5, 93
Psychometric theories, 153

Qualitative comments, 56, 84–86, 156, 160, 192

Qualitative data, 143, 154, 159, 159, 164
Quality assurance, vii, xii, 78, 143, 158, 159, 159, 161, 162, 164, 197
Quantitative data, 32, 143, 144, 154, 160

Rating scale, 15, 16, 85, 86, 137, 139, 140, 160, 178, 181, 188, 192, 194
Real patient, vi, viii, 2, 3, 5, 6, 11, 16, 18, 19, 68, 93, 94, 96–104, 106, 109, 111–113, 172, 193
Realism, 94, 96, 97, 106, 109, 110, 112, 113, 118, 119
Reliability, 19, 23, 24, 27, 28, 30, 31, 34, 77, 78, 81, 95, 122, 125, 131, 144, 147, 148, 153, 154, 182, 184, 189, 190, 194
Remediation, xi, 104, 160, 165–167, 169–175, 197
Reproducibility, xi, 104, 165–167, 169–175, 197

Sampling strategy, 23, 28, 30, 31
Scaling, 161
Scoring template, 28, 66, 77, 78, 81, 83–85, 87, 90, 96, 106, 156, 161
Security, 75, 130, 162, 195
Selection OSCE, 177, 178–186
Short case, 2, 9, 15, 17–19

Short station, 190
Shows how, 9–12, 18, 20, 21,
    183, 184
Simulated patient, vi, 5, 6, 19,
    59, 66, 68, 69, 76, 93–101,
    104–106, 109–113, 118,
    124, 155, 157, 162, 178,
    192, 193
Simulation, vi, vii, 5, 6, 73,
    101, 110–112, 116, 173
Simulator, 6, 73, 93, 94, 105,
    109–119
Situational judgement test,
    180
Specificity, 14, 17
Standard setting, v, vii, 78, 128,
    133–138, 140, 142, 181,
    195
Standardization, 5, 6, 18, 20,
    94–96, 101, 103, 106, 112,
    122, 166, 168

Standardized patient, vi, vii, 5,
    6, 19, 27, 34, 35, 66–68, 72,
    74, 76, 93, 94, 97, 100, 109,
    112, 117, 118, 123–125,
    172, 192, 197
Static station, 56, 57
Summative OSCE, 55, 56, 109,
    118, 128, 142, 192, 195,
    197

Threats to validity, 25

Utility, 23, 34, 177, 182

Validity, vi, viii, 19, 21, 23–26,
    28, 30, 31, 34, 37, 38, 54,
    77, 82, 83, 95, 96, 131, 182,
    184, 189, 190

AUTHORS' BIOGRAPHIES

Hamza Mohammad Abdulghani
MBBS, DPHC, ABFM, FRCGP (UK), Masters in Medical
Education (MMEdu)
Associate Professor of Family Medicine
Head of the Assessment and Evaluation Unit
College of Medicine, King Saud University, Riyadh, Saudi Arabia

Dr. Abdulghani is an educationist and family physician with a special interest in assessment. Prior to joining the Medical Education Department, King Saud University Medical College, Saudi Arabia, he had organized and conducted many faculty development workshops for medical schools. Dr. Abdulghani has established the centralized assessment system in the College. He has been a member of the Examination Committee for the Postgraduate Family Medicine Program of the Saudi Commission for Health Specialties since its inception in 1997. He serves as a consultant for many newly established medical colleges and an external examiner for different medical colleges' undergraduate and postgraduate programs. Dr. Abdulghani's consultations and workshops have focused on clinical teaching and learning, feedback skills, and different types of assessment. His current research interests include the development and improvement of an assessment system that produces innovative, more valid, and reliable test materials.

Gominda Ponnamperuma
MBBS, Dip. Psychology, Masters in the Medical Education
(MMEd), PhD
Senior Lecturer in Medical Education, Faculty of Medicine,
University of Colombo, Sri Lanka

Dr Ponnamperuma has served as a resource person in many international symposia, conferences, and workshops. He has authored many journal articles, book chapters, and books. He is an editorial board member of the journals *Medical Education Online* and *BMC Medical Education*. A tutor, examiner, and resource material developer for national and international medical education courses, Dr. Ponnamperuma has also carried out consultations for educational projects. His research interests include assessment (including selection for training) and curriculum development and evaluation.

Zubair Amin
MBBS; Diplomat, the American Board of Pediatrics; Masters in
Health Profession Education (MHPE)
Associate Professor of Pediatrics, Yong Loo Lin School of Medicine,
National University of Singapore

Senior Consultant, Department of Neonatology, National
University Hospital, Singapore

Dr. Amin is an Associate Professor in the Department of Pediatrics, National University of Singapore, and Senior Consultant Neonatologist at National University Hospital, Singapore. His immediate past appointments include Deputy Head, Medical Education Unit, National University of Singapore. He also served as Assistant Dean for Curriculum and Assessment at the School of Medicine. He is the lead author/editor of three books: *Basics in Medical Education (2nd edition)*; *Profiles of Asian Medical Schools: Part I Southeast Asia*; and *Practical Guide to Medical Student Assessment*. He is the recipient of the University Teaching Excellence Award (2006) and the Friends of the Medical Students Award (2008) by the Medical Society, National University of Singapore. Dr. Amin has conducted numerous workshops and staff development programs on assessment, evaluation, and the OSCE in Asia, Europe, the Middle-east and Africa. His interests are in assessment, faculty development, and international medical education.

www.ingramcontent.com/pod-product-compliance
Lightning Source LLC
Chambersburg PA
CBHW061248220326
41599CB00028B/5571